Save Your Life *Now*

Your Health is in Your Hands

Save Your Life *Now*

Dr. April Schulte
DAOM, LAc

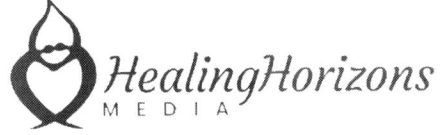

Copyright 2019 by Healing Horizons Media. All rights reserved.
No part of this book may be reproduced, stored in a retrieval system, or transmitted by any means, electronic, mechanical, photocopy, recording, or otherwise, without written permission from the author.

ISBN: 978-1-7336167-0-6
eISBN: 978-1-7336167-1-3

Printed in the United States of America

Editor: Jessica Vineyard, Red Letter Editing, LLC
www.redletterediting.com
Cover and interior design: Constellation Book Services

This book is dedicated to each and every patient I have had the honor of serving in my career. I feel so blessed to share my gifts of healing with them, and in return, I have learned and continue to learn so much from them.

Contents

Foreword	ix
Preface	xiii
Acknowledgments	xxi
Introduction	1
Chapter 1. Why Conventional Medicine Alone Does Not Work	3
Chapter 2. The Mind, Body, and Spirit Connection	19
Chapter 3. Traditional Chinese Medicine	25
Chapter 4. Benefits of Integrative and Collaborative Medicine	45
Chapter 5. Key Therapies in Integrative and Collaborative Medicine	57
Chapter 6. Your Emotions and Your Health	83
Chapter 7. Climbing Out of a Health Hole	95
Chapter 8. Digestion, the Center of Health	99
Chapter 9. Finding the Delicate Balance to Achieving Optimal Health	107
Chapter 10. Snapshots of Integrated Health Solutions	115
Chapter 11. Take Back Your Health Care Power	125
Chapter 12. The Staggering Costs of Health Care	133
Chapter 13. A Dying Patient's Perspective on Integrated Health Solutions	135
Index	145

Foreword

One of the most memorable papers I wrote during my doctoral training was about spirit. I wrote it in 1980, a few weeks after my two-year-old daughter died, when my spirit felt so broken that I was not sure it would ever heal. Not only was my spirit greatly suffering, but so were my mind and body. I either cried for a good part of each day or was almost catatonic. My body ached and felt bruised. This was the first time I had a clear and personal experience with how the mind, body, and spirit are intimately intertwined.

After I healed (although a small, vulnerable spot remained in my heart), I reflected on the fact that every part of my being had been profoundly affected by the loss of my daughter. This recognition led me to begin a study of mind-body health, which continued through many years of teaching and applying the concepts to patients in my practice. I am now a psychologist and health and life coach and am fully integrated into Dr. April Schulte's integrative and collaborative complementary care clinic, and every day I feel blessed to be part of this amazing practice.

I was fortunate in my early training to attend live workshops with the likes of Andrew Weil, Deepak Chopra, Jon Kabat-Zinn, Candace Pert, Martin Rossman, and David Bresler, all of whom are influential leaders in the changing face of health practices. Following their lead, medical and psychological research is now studying health and not just disease.

Weil suggested in his 1983 book *Health and Healing* that standard medical practice ignored consciousness as a determinant of health and encouraged a different understanding. Chopra, in his book *The Healing Self*, brought forth one of the first arguments for the fact that there is no separation between the mind and body, that what happens in one immediately effects the other. Rossman, a pioneer in imagery work, says in his book *Guided Imagery for Self-Healing*, "You were born with the ability to heal. [You can learn] to use your mind to fully utilize your innate healing power." Modern research has confirmed these ideas about mind-body medicine. All problems, whether initially presenting with emotional symptoms or physical, are, in actuality, both.

Dr. Schulte and I have been colleagues and friends for almost ten years. In that time, I have seen how she is both a visionary and a doer. In this engaging and timely book, she describes how complementary and integrative medicine can be a vital part of the healing journey.

As with my journey, Dr. Schulte's personal health challenges led her to a deep personal understanding of the connections between mind, body, and spirit. She found that it took a whole team of health care practitioners to return her to health, and she eventually realized what was missing: a guide who held a roadmap to recovery. She has since become that guide, and this book is one of the roadmaps she has created to share her experience, wisdom, and insights with the wider public. Her desire is to encourage people to understand themselves as whole humans and to educate them about taking charge of their health.

Dr. Schulte is a true pioneer in mind-body health and is deeply committed to her vision of a better way to treat patients. This vision, coupled with her willingness to take action, has led her to bring together a talented team of practitioners from a variety of health care specialties. I have personally witnessed my patients (and myself) experience the synergy that occurs when various treatment modalities come together and prove that treating the whole person is far more effective than any individual treatment alone.

Traditional Chinese Medicine (TCM) holds a profound respect for the mind-body-spirit connection that is central to all TCM treatments. Dr. Schulte's specialized training in TCM taught her to look at disease, illness, and pain with a perspective different from that of traditional Western medicine. Consequently, she encourages patients to look beyond traditional Western medicine to find the deeper causes of their disease, pain, or disorder.

Dr. Schulte is a leader and a guide, always reminding patients that they are unique and deserving of a thoughtful, in-depth assessment and treatment of their issues. If your health matters to you, and I am sure it does, especially since you decided to pick up this book, then I encourage you to be mindful of the words of wisdom and insights Dr. Schulte provides here. We believe you have a right to make health choices that fit your beliefs and values, that it is up to you to take charge of your health and ask for what you want. Do not settle for less.

I hope that you will be encouraged and motivated by the information contained in this book and that you will be inspired to take action on behalf of your own health.

Paula King, PhD
Psychologist, Health and Life Coach
Author, *A Trust Walk: Mindful Golf*
Grand Junction, CO

Preface

When I was twelve years old, my dissatisfaction with the narrow-mindedness of conventional Western medicine became personal. I was in the throes of hormonal instability and was training intensely to one day become a professional dancer. My body was changing in so many ways and so quickly that I was emotionally and physically miserable. I was desperate for help as my emotions took me on a rollercoaster ride almost daily, my menstrual cycles were tremendously painful, and my right hip hurt so badly that it completely disrupted my normal daily living.

When I sought help from our family's primary care physician as a pre-teen, his answers did not satisfy me. "You have menstrual cramps and mood swings. Just take birth control." "Your hip hurts? Just stop putting your leg by your ear." I thought, *Um . . . no thank you. My body has hormonal imbalances that need to be addressed at the root of the problem, not covered up by a drug. I live to dance [which to this day involves putting my leg by my ear], so there must be another solution.*

In college and away from the support of my family, I caved in and tried birth control, as my menstrual cramps had become even more horrendous. The medication created such horrific side effects that I did not recognize myself. I discontinued the drug and sought other answers, which would take me years to find. In spite of my physical and hormonal suffering, I achieved my dream of dancing professionally, but with that dream came the development of multiple eating disorders.

As it turns out, my internal wisdom at the age of twelve was right, but I did not find meaningful answers for my health issues until fifteen years later, when I realized there were actual solutions to my emotional mood swings, my painful periods, my hip pain, and my eating disorders, but they would not come easily. In fact, I like to say that it took a village to get me better.

Finding appropriate answers for achieving a healthful state of homeostasis involved a focused care plan that addressed my health mentally, emotionally, physically, and spiritually. As a patient suffering from debilitating diseases who also had a passion for medicine and the healing arts, I began to make the connections between how each modality of care was helpful to me and how the integration of therapies amplified the positive effects. I also saw gaps in the continuity of care because my health care practitioners were not collaborating and working as a team. I was left to draw the map quest for achieving my best possible health myself.

It was then that I had a professional epiphany. I realized I was blessed to be interested enough about health to heal myself. I thought, *What if I had not had an interest in the intricacies of figuring out how to navigate my own health care? What if anatomy, physiology, endocrinology, neurology, pharmacology, and psychology had eluded me—not to mention trying to figure out how complementary medicine could fit into the picture? What about the people who are as desperate as I was to feel better?*

As an intern at the Oregon College of Oriental Medicine, one of my first patients helped me realize the importance of partnership between practitioner and patient. This patient was a twenty-year-old female with the chief complaint of diarrhea with mucous. My fellow intern and I recommended, as part of a comprehensive treatment plan, to discontinue eating cheese after she admitted her symptoms were worse after eating the food. The patient refused to follow our recommendation, and I remember thinking, *Well, enjoy your mucous-filled diarrhea.*

That experience made an impression on me. Patients who expected a magic wand to be waved over them to bring them to a state of optimal health would not be comfortable with me as a healer. While gifted healers may seem magical, as their patients can get better under their care, the healing process is not magical. It requires an effort from both patient and practitioner alike.

Toward the end of my master's-level training, I was already contemplating who I wanted to be for my patients and the level of care I wanted to provide. I had developed the belief that a healing process is most efficient as a partnership between practitioner and patient. This would especially hold true with those patients who had not found successful treatment elsewhere.

Between graduating with my master's degree in Traditional Chinese Medicine (TCM) in Oregon and getting my license established in Colorado, I took the time to develop a business plan for an acupuncture and TCM herbal practice. I knew that the name and logo I chose would set the tone for the very nature of my business.

Shortly after I graduated, I packed up my Volkswagen Jetta and began the long drive across the open prairies toward my home in Grand Junction, Colorado. Looking at the horizon as I drove mile after mile, the name for my business came to me: "Healing Horizons."

I knew that it was the responsibility of patients to take proactive steps to achieve their desired health goals. I also knew that it would be my responsibility as a healer to teach, guide, provide healing treatments, and remind them of their own healing potential. I wanted these main conceptualizations of my practice exemplified by my logo. One day, while perusing the side streets of Seaside, Oregon, I spotted a statue in the window of a store. As soon as I saw it, I felt it encompassed the partnership between practitioner and patient, so I snapped a picture of it. I had no extra money back then to purchase the statue. Later, this image became the basis from which my graphic designer worked to design my business logo. The figure is seen on the cover of this book and at the beginning of each chapter. Two figures form a figure eight and symbolize the patient and practitioner working together in a harmonious partnership. In Chinese culture, the number eight is thought to embody good luck and prosperity. It was a perfect match!

The Birth of Healing Horizons Integrated Health Solutions

My healing approach of utilizing the collaboration and integration of therapies evolved as I worked to create a successful health clinic called Healing Horizons Integrated Health Solutions in the beautiful desert area of southwest Colorado, in my hometown of Grand Junction. The red rocks and painted desert provide a beautiful landscape for amazing healing to occur for its people. The story of how I created the health clinic demonstrates the framework for which I developed this highly efficient method of achieving and maintaining health.

I have had an interest in health since I was a little girl. My grandmother and my mother shared an interest in natural medicine, and I followed suit. As I grew up, I loved studying the human body. As an undergraduate, I could not keep my nose out of anatomy and physiology, biochemistry, endocrinology, and genetic text books. In my post-graduate work, my interests expanded to include more complementary medicine therapies when my sights were cracked open by studying Traditional Chinese Medicine. However, my first tried-

and-true experience of thinking about health from a collaborative and integrative health care view occurred as I faced and conquered one of my biggest health challenges.

It would start with a gnawing feeling in my stomach that would occur immediately the moment I lifted a fork to my mouth: a feeling of disgust swirled with fear. The act of eating would heighten my senses so strongly that I could "feel" my fat; I thought I could literally feel my fat cells swelling in my abdomen and thighs. These haunting thoughts would consume me until I purged the food, at which time I would experience significant relief. Sometimes I would repeat the entire cycle of eating, feeling miserable for having done so, and purging as many as twenty times a day. Relatively few people know the insides of toilet bowls like I do.

At the time, the only connection I could make between food and my body was that food could make the feeling of my fat cells swelling worse. My battle with bulimia addiction came after a long stint of severe food restriction that coincided with over-exercise. These habits were greatly exacerbated by the rigors of being in show business, in which a perfect "dancer's body" was expected and demanded by my producers. Because of my eating disorders, in my late twenties, I experienced what it likely feels like to go into menopause and for my organs to do their mightiest to keep going without having proper nourishment. Without nutrients to serve as building blocks to support my metabolism, hormone regulation, immune system, and more, my health was quickly spiraling downward. Once I decided I was going to get better, I entered a mental, emotional, physical, and spiritual journey back to being healthy.

Today, I am blessed to report that my health has improved tremendously. What finally motivated me to resolve my disordered eating addiction was my deep desire to live in what I had come to know as my purpose, which was to be a healer. I knew that each time I threw up in the toilet or denied my body the nourishment and building blocks it needed to function with strength and ease, I would be that much further away from living my life's purpose. I knew it would take incredible internal strength, sheer will, and support from those closest to me to regain my health.

There was no magic bullet that helped me, but instead, a synergy of therapies coincided with changes in habits to help me heal. I knew I wanted to avoid pharmaceutical medications, so I sought acupuncture, homeopathy, chiropractic, counseling, life coaching, Chinese herbs, massage, functional medicine, and other treatments. I began to experience how each modality of care helped me in different ways and that the total benefit from all of the modalities working together was greater than the sum of the parts. For example, when I changed my negative thinking patterns and associated behaviors, my body responded better to the other modalities, which in turn helped give me more energy, improved my mental and emotional states, normalized my digestive function, and strengthened my immune system.

Throughout my healing process, I experienced what it is like to be a sick patient who wants to get better and has to take on the daunting task of navigating the health care system. I had to make the connects between my symptoms and the different modalities I used and orchestrate collaboration between my practitioners. It seemed obvious to me that my practitioners would communicate with one another to help efficiently guide my healing process, but it didn't happen.

I had developed a model of health care for my own healing that I came to realize would work well for others. It was then that my intention to create a truly collaborative and integrative medicine clinic was born. I created the healing center with a team of caring health care professionals who appreciate the value of considering the unique health care needs of each individual patient and who address patients' chief complaints methodically and thoroughly by utilizing the best of what each modality of care has to offer. I have learned that combining various therapies creates a synergy from which the healing potential of each modality is enhanced by the addition of the other.

Our bodies desire and are magnificently programmed to be healthy. However, by the time we have developed symptoms of an illness, there are layers of emotional, physical, and mental imbalances to sort through. There is often a spiritual component, as well. (I use the term "spiritual" to reflect the unique belief system of each patient.) It is vitally important to accept that in order to achieve and maintain health, no one single change you make, no one medication, person, or any one thing will take you down a path of true healing. True healing requires your commitment and your team of practitioners to delve deeply into the root causes of the imbalance, whether it presents physically, mentally, or emotionally, and address each one appropriately.

As for me, I am so much better, yet the journey continues. I am aware of the importance of continuing self-care to help my mind, body, and spirit work in alignment with one another. As a doctor of acupuncture and Oriental medicine and owner and clinic director of a successful complementary integrative medicine practice, I now know the importance of patients choosing health care options that align with their value systems.

I am passionate about reaching as many people as possible with my message by taking the "woo-woo" out of complementary medicine approaches such as acupuncture, chiropractic, massage, homeopathy, functional medicine, and other therapies. It is important to meet patients where they are in their knowledge and belief systems, because their health matters. *Your* health matters. It is time to save your life *now*.

Acknowledgments

To my husband, Kevin, thank you for your unwavering love for me and sharing in my commitment and passion for integrative and collaborative medicine. To my children, Adam and RubyJean, thank you for motivating me to be a better person. To my mother, Kathryn, father (in heaven), Terry, and my sisters Crystal and Rachel, thank you for your love and relentless support. To my colleagues, thank you for continuing to feed my spirit as we forge forward as pioneers in understanding and developing the power of integrative and collaborative medicine. A special thank you to each and every teacher I have had in my life. My deepest appreciation goes to each of you for your commitment to education.

Introduction

Have you been bouncing from doctor to doctor and from website to website in search of a solution for a lingering health problem? Are you desperate to get some long-term relief and to reestablish your health? If so, the information in this book holds the roadmap to health you have been looking for.

I wrote this book to share the solutions I have found as a complementary integrative health practitioner. This method has worked for thousands of my patients as well as my own health challenges. The information here will deliver a totally different approach to achieving your health goals in a way that is easy to understand. Using this truly integrative approach to treat and manage your health concerns, from chronic pain to autoimmune conditions, will give you the results you have always wanted.

Save Your Life Now: Your Health is in Your Hands provides a general framework in which to think about and successfully address your health and how to take your health care power back. Examples of health conditions I have effectively treated using this integrated method of care

are provided, and patient stories and testimonials are given throughout the book to give you hope that you, too, can feel great again.

Please note that the term "healing team," used throughout the book, is defined as a patient and his or her team of health care practitioners who work together to achieve health goals as set forth by the patient.

Since you picked up this book, you are likely dissatisfied with the state of your current health and perhaps have a sense of unease about the health care you have received.

It is my hope that you will read this book and feel inspired to take charge of your health now and to feel empowered not to settle for the status quo offered by our current health care model. Learning that our physical, mental, emotional, and spiritual health is interconnected opens up options of care you may not have otherwise considered for achieving your health goals. Your health is in your hands. You can take your health care power back and make choices that are perfect for you to facilitate your healing journey.

CHAPTER 1
Why Conventional Medicine Alone Does Not Work

Conventional Western medicine has a lot to offer health care consumers. I can speak to that professionally and personally. As a doctor of acupuncture and Oriental medicine and a leader in the collaborative and integrative approach to health care, I value conventional Western medicine for several reasons. The diagnostics provided by imaging studies and blood work are excellent tools for assessing what is going on with a patient, and I regularly consider such diagnostics to guide my advice, both within my scope of practice and to make referrals to practitioners outside of it. It is occasionally necessary to combine my treatment methods with those of conventional Western medicine, and I have sometimes advised my patients to talk with their allopathic doctors regarding other options. I regularly collaborate with these doctors regarding integrating a patient's care.

It is an honor to work alongside conventional Western medical doctors in a concerted effort to help our mutual patients achieve wellness. There have been plenty of times in my professional career that I did not want to see a patient if he or she were not also under the care of conventional Western medical doctors. I have even had the occasion to refuse care to patients who did not first seek the care of a medical doctor. I have medical doctors as my patients and accept referrals from and collaborate with them. I respect the positive aspects of what conventional Western medicine has to offer.

Conventional Western medicine has even been a huge blessing for me and my family. If it weren't for modern medicine, my husband and I would not have been able to conceive our twins, and even if we had, the twins and I would have probably died in the delivery process without it.

During my pregnancy, I developed a condition called HELLP syndrome, in which my liver and kidneys started to fail, my platelets plummeted, and my blood pressure skyrocketed. At thirty-four weeks of pregnancy (six weeks short of full term), I was told the babies would be delivered via emergency C-section. I was knocked out for the emergency surgery, as I would likely bleed out. Remarkably, I did not. I was placed on a magnesium sulfate drip, which made me very weak. Meanwhile, the twins were probed with wires and needles and feeding tubes in the neonatal intensive care unit. When I finally met my babies the day after their birth, I was so exhausted and sick that I could barely hold them. When I did hold them for the first time, it was only for a few minutes. Then the nurses untangled the cords between us to take them back so I could rest.

While conventional Western medicine saved my life and the lives of my twins, it failed me in my return back to health from HELLP syndrome. (Conventional medicine does not know what causes the syndrome.) I was alive but still sick and had symptoms that could not be explained or treated by conventional medicine, so my conventional medical doctors offered limited guidance on how to get well.

Fortunately for me and my family, I had the wisdom to seek my own team of health care practitioners to restore my health. I sought the care of acupuncturists, chiropractors, massage therapists, a counselor and psychologist, a homeopath, and a functional medicine practitioner to create my path back to feeling like my vibrant and healthy self.

Many conventional Western medicine doctors have no idea what these complementary therapies can do to help their patients. It is rare to find a medical doctor who honors, respects, and values the inherent qualities that come from bringing such therapies together for the better good of their patients, though they are certainly out there. Patients regularly report simple tolerance from their doctors toward the idea of complementary care. Every once in a while, I even hear about a doctor who is adamantly opposed to complementary treatment methods. I believe this is because of the nature of medical training our doctors receive in the conventional Western medical model. In our current health care system, little recognition is given to the fact that a whole system exists in each person that acts cooperatively, reactively, and synergistically to affect health. Applying this knowledge in Western medicine is even rarer.

When conventional Western medicine is at a loss to make a suitable diagnosis and corresponding treatment plan, then doctors who provide complementary therapies have an advantage when patients seek their help. This is because more obvious causes for disease have been ruled out by conventional medicine testing, allowing the complementary care practitioner to operate more comfortably within each paradigm offered by the respective modality of care. As a healer and someone who knows there are viable options for achieving optimal health, I worry about the millions of people who stop at options provided solely by conventional Western medicine. Too often patients limit themselves in their healing capacity by resolving to take a medication prescribed by their doctor that often causes a long list of side effects, which can then lead to further imbalances, disease, and chronic illness.

Quite often, the patients who need the most help are the ones who limit themselves to the care provided by their primary care doctors. For example, patients who have been labeled with an incurable disease diagnosis or those who feel terrible but whose conventional medical doctors cannot find out why are likely to fall prey to the dangerous idea that feeling unwell is what they can expect for the rest of their lives. It doesn't have to be this way. It is time we open our minds to the possibilities of health and healing outside of conventional medicine. Our health care system needs help, and we the people can take our health care power back.

Top Reasons Patients Are Dissatisfied with Conventional Medicine

It is important to identify what is not working in our standard health care system to appreciate the benefits of integrating mind, body, and spirit in the form of integrative and collaborative care. I have learned from conversations with my patient base that there are five primary reasons why patients are not satisfied with the conventional care they typically receive.

REASON #1: PHARMACEUTICAL DRUGS

The first line of defense against most symptoms and diseases is a pharmaceutical drug. According to Statista, a website that aggregates statistics and studies from thousands of sources, the US pharmaceutical industry is the "world's most important national market." In 2016, the top three pharmaceutical companies generated 72 billion dollars of profit on pharmaceuticals alone.*

We have been trained to think that there is a drug to match nearly every symptom and disease. Pharmaceutical companies capitalize on this every day, which is demonstrated by the millions of dollars they spend annually to promote their drugs in TV commercials. It seems they have drugs to cure almost anything that ails you. While the commercials match symptoms and diseases with specific drugs, they must also disclose, by law, potential side effects as mild as weight gain, diarrhea, and tremors and as severe as organ failure and death. Meanwhile,

---

* Statista: The Statistics Portal, https://www.statista.com/.

they hope your emotional response to the visual cues in the commercials of happy people dancing through fields of daisies will distract you from the reality of the listed side effects, the results of which will likely ensue once you start using the drug.

Despite the fact that there are innumerable potential side effects to these drugs ranging from fatigue and nausea to death, they are just one downside to taking a pharmaceutical drug by matching it to a symptom or disease. The bigger problem is that the drug rarely cures the patient. Instead, it often inhibits the body's natural ability to heal itself, thereby leading to further imbalances and disease.

While pharmaceutical intervention certainly can and does serve a purpose, medications tend to rob people of learning to listen to the clues their bodies give to show that their systems are out of balance. As humans, we are in a constant state of flux influenced by our emotions, physical health, spiritual health, our environment, and other factors, and our emotional, mental, and physical symptoms are there to guide us. If these cues are muted or changed as a result of taking a medication, it is easier to get caught off the health track. Your power lies in thinking beyond the option of medications for a symptom or disease, even when your doctor does not know other options.

REASON #2: BOXED-IN THINKING

Most medical doctors are not trained to think beyond the conventional Western medicine model. The fact that most medical doctors are not trained to consider options outside of conventional Western medicine has become a source of vexation for many complementary care providers and patients alike. In general, the health care system is set up to look at microsystems and ignore the macrosystem. Rarely are treatment plans developed with the idea of supporting the whole person from head to toe. Sometimes it is apparent that the words to the song I learned in elementary school, "The hip bone's connected to the knee bone, the knee bone's connected to the ankle bone," are not even considered. There are a myriad of things to think about to determine which plan of action is best for the well-being of the whole patient.

There is a common analogy that managing our health is like maintaining a car. Both our bodies and our cars require regular maintenance. However, the similarities end there. Conventional Western medicine views health similarly to how a mechanic thinks about fixing a car. If a car part is broken, the mechanic fixes or replaces the part. While this method works well for fixing cars, it does not work well for the healing of human beings. Unfortunately, our current health care model emulates the method of care for car maintenance rather than considering that the human body is dynamic. For example, in our current health care system, common logic for treatment is as follows: Is something wrong with the lungs? Treat the lungs. Is the patient experiencing stomach pain? Treat the stomach. Is something wrong with the emotions? Prescribe an antidepressant. Is the patient experiencing acid reflux? Recommend an acid blocker. Does the patient have pain? Give a painkiller. Does the patient have high cholesterol? Prescribe a statin. Is the gallbladder inflamed? Well, just take it out.

In conventional medicine, the human body is identified as and treated by its individual parts; rarely is it treated as an integrated whole. Specialists in conventional medicine focus on only one specific system, organ, or body part. These doctors end up knowing a whole lot about that specific area of medicine but have relatively little idea of how that particular part of the body affects or is affected by the rest of the system.

This way of practicing medicine is called a "reductionist" view of health. We have become so wrapped up in the breaking down of parts and studying them that our current thinking about health separates each cell, each organ, each hormonal gland, and each nerve from the rest of the system. In reality, each and every cell, organ, hormonal gland, and nerve work harmoniously together—that is the inherent goal, anyway—and cannot be separated from the others.

Our health is not meant to be plugged into a one-size-fits-all system of matching specific symptoms to specific treatment protocols. It is important to take responsibility for your own health, especially as a patient, and to know that covering up or ignoring your symptoms will only wreak further havoc in your system. One of the best ways to take charge of your own health care is to ask your health care practitioners to look deeper for answers to your health concerns.

REASON #3: THE LIMITS OF SCIENCE

There is too much emphasis on respecting only that which is scientific. I respect science; I even love science because it sheds light on the unknowns of our world and our bodies. I grew up studying the basics of the scientific method, which would become the framework for my entire pre-med program as an undergraduate.

Looking back, I felt comfortable studying science because it provided a relatively simple and concrete perspective of the world we live in. I felt a quiet yet profound trust in knowing that while science was complicated, it was black and white. Scientific facts are either true or false. However, I became so immersed in learning all of the micro-facts about various subjects, from pharmacology and endocrinology to molecular genetics, that I got lost in the minutia, and the bigger picture of health escaped me.

I would not know that I had gotten lost until later in my life, when I studied and then began practicing TCM. I now fully understand that when science reveals another truth, it opens so many other doors of possibility into how the body works that it supports the adage, "The more you know, the more you don't know." This concept is uncomfortable for many scientists.

Science provides a framework from which to attempt to understand the world and our bodies in the world; there is so much more to understand than we do now. In fact, there are so many unknowns about our universe and our bodies that it is silly to use only what we do know as scientific proof to find wellness. While medical research remains our greatest tool to discovering the truth behind science, it is still quite limited and presents challenges to studying complementary medical therapies.

For example, the gold standard of medical research—double-blind, randomized control trials—and the resulting evidence may be well applied to many medical interventions. However, applying this method of research to TCM and other complementary methods of care is like trying to fit a square peg into a round hole. It is unrealistic to try to squeeze centuries-old holistic therapies into the current rigors of medical research, which has been designed to look at specific and limited outcomes.

Usually, in randomized control trials, research is focused on one variable, such as a drug, procedure, or an objective measure of a specific outcome or biological marker, but isolating specific variables changes the very nature of how medicine is meant to be practiced. TCM practitioners are likely to make several TCM diagnoses where conventional Western medicine practitioners would make only a single disease diagnosis. Furthermore, they expect several outcomes from a treatment plan created for an individual patient.

The fields of TCM and integrative medicine are challenged in getting research funding. While the National Institutes of Health and the National Center for Complementary and Alternative Medicine do fund research, the overall budget is relatively small. Ideally, research methods that are conducive to both conventional and integrative medicine would provide a holistic approach that would benefit patients. In other words, more research would be done that incorporates TCM differential diagnoses of patients with conventional medicine diagnoses.

According to an article in the journal *Complementary Therapies in Medicine*, whole-systems research is being developed to measure "a whole package of care" from which practitioners can look at a set of treatments and a whole range of clinical outcomes based on the idea of treating multiple symptoms through an integrative treatment approach.*

REASON #4: DEPENDENCE ON CONVENTIONAL MEDICINE TEST RESULTS

Conventional Western medicine is dependent on abnormalities found in lab work and imaging studies to make a diagnosis and treatment plan. Having been trained in and being dependent on concrete signs and symptoms that match a disease diagnosis, doctors of conventional Western medicine are reliant on objective measures found in blood work and imaging studies to form a concrete diagnosis. Subjective measures, or the patient's description of symptoms, are sometimes considered, but a certain rubric, or statement of purpose, has to apply before a diagnosis can be made. From that diagnosis, a treatment plan is considered.

However, if a diagnosis is not made, as is often the case when a patient has a variety of symptoms but lab work and imaging studies come back normal, Western medicine is often at a loss, leaving the doctor with limited options for treatment. Unfortunately, this is when antidepressants, antibiotics, and painkillers are often and hastily prescribed with the mere hope that they will help.

A shortfall in conventional Western medicine is its dependence on labeling to identify a disease in order to establish a treatment plan. Since the tools available to conventional treatment usually involve pharmaceutical drugs (of which there is one available for most any disease diagnosis), doctors are limited and often do not think outside of the pharmaceutical box for ways to help their patients.

Too often, movement toward helping a patient feel better is postponed until a diagnosis is found, which perpetuates disease progression. There

---

* MJ Verhoef, G. Lewith, C. Ritenbaugh, et al., "Complementary and Alternative Medicine Whole Systems Research: Beyond Identification of Inadequacies of the RCT," *Complementary Therapies in Medicine*, vol. 13 (3): Sept 2005, p. 206–212.

is always something that can be done while a diagnosis is being sought. Why wait before trying therapies outside of conventional Western medicine to find answers and relief? Your health asks you to take responsibility for seeking many sources of health care.

REASON #5: LIMITED INSURANCE COVERAGE
Insurance doesn't always cover treatments that will actually help a patient. We are a society focused on sick care, and nearly all health care providers get paid when they provide care for sick people. Imagine a health care system in which health care professionals are paid when their patients are well instead of when they are sick. How might our health and health care expenses be different?

Pharmaceutical companies make many millions of dollars by selling medications to sick people. While there are times when conventional medications are necessary, there are plenty of times when patients can avoid taking medications by simply choosing a different route of care. Instead of relying on health insurance coverage, consider alternative strategies for financially preparing to manage your health. For example, several of my patients use health savings accounts. Also, consider that investing in health maintenance by receiving regular complementary treatments will save you illness and therefore time and money down the road. When you take measures to prevent illness, you increase your chances of not needing conventional Western medical interventions.

Preventive Medicine

The American College of Preventive Medicine defines preventive medicine as health care that "focuses on the health of individuals, communities, and defined populations . . . [with the goal to] protect, promote, and maintain health and well-being and to prevent disease, disability, and death."* Unfortunately, typical conventional medicine preventive measures often do not reach deep enough into the root causes of disease.

Preventive medicine does not mean catching a disease in its early stages; it mean keeping people well and involves patient education on what keeps the mind, body, and spirit thriving. Therefore, while tests such as mammograms, blood draws, and annual exams may be helpful to find disease early, they are still focused on sick care. This is where my appreciation and deep sense of respect for TCM comes in. Despite operating in a society in which most folks seek care when they are sick, TCM is rooted in the concept of true preventive medicine.

A patient coming to a TCM practitioner to maintain wellness is a celebratory moment because he or she has opened doors to considering options outside of conventional medicine. The patient will be exposed to new ideas about health, which will greatly expand treatment options for both the chief complaint of the moment and health concerns in the future. TCM uses objective measures such as tongue and pulse readings to pick up on lurking imbalances and then reestablishes balance in the system before the patient gets symptoms and becomes ill. If we used therapies such as TCM as a standard approach to care, people would become less sick and less often, thereby avoiding expensive disease treatments.

I recognize more and more that patients in my practice desire true answers to their health concerns. For this to happen, it is important that patients and health care practitioners alike consider that each patient is a unique individual and that symptoms in one part of the body are rarely isolated from other parts. For example, a patient who is suffering from the deteriorating health of one organ system may be effectively treated by first attending to a supportive organ system. Our organs (and all other tissues) are connected in more ways than science

---

* American College of Preventive Medicine, "Preventive Medicine," https://www.acpm.org/page/preventivemedicine.

can show, and they work together and are dependent on one another. Thus, treating only the diseased organ does not always work. It is appropriate for patient and healer to look deeper into the system.

The connections in the body are endless because we are not whole beings composed of individual parts; rather, we are whole beings for which one part is not separate from another. The health of our cells, organs, emotions, mind, and spirit indeed are dependent on the body operating as one magnificent system.

The nervous, hormonal, and circulatory systems; organs; and other tissues of the body work together like a well-oiled and finely tuned machine. When a symptom appears, it is a sign that something elsewhere in the system is off balance. Symptoms are the body's way of providing clues to find the root cause of an imbalance that needs to be addressed. When symptoms are ignored, the body talks louder and louder in the form of exacerbated symptoms until the patient is forced to listen.

Say that ten patients present with a chief complaint of elbow pain. Their primary care doctors would diagnose all of them as having the common affliction of lateral epicondylitis, commonly known as tennis elbow or elbow tendonitis. Practitioners practicing from an integrative care perspective, however, would diagnose each patient individually by looking at each one's entire health picture.

The elbow is not an isolated structure within the body, which is why treating only the elbow is usually not the best treatment plan to yield the most positive outcome. The elbow joint is made of bones, cartilage, synovial fluid, and tendons, with surrounding connective tissues such as fascia and ligaments. It is also directly connected to the wrist and shoulder joints. While this may be as obvious as "the neck bone is connected to the back bone," there is more to it. Structurally, if one joint becomes impaired in its ability to function optimally, other joints and surrounding connective tissues may also be impaired; there is usually more to tendonitis than the musculoskeletal system.

Let's consider one way tendonitis may be associated with other imbalances deeper in the system. After taking a complete review of systems, from which the practitioner gains a general understanding of how the patient's body is functioning, the practitioner realizes that the patient's digestive system is compromised. This is conveyed by symptoms such as acid reflux, excess gas or bloating after eating, and alternating diarrhea and constipation.

From a Traditional Chinese Medicine perspective, this weakened digestive state leads to blood deficiency. In TCM, blood has several primary functions, one of which is nourishing the soft connective tissues of the body, especially tendons. However, determining there is a digestive weakness is not the ending point, either. It is important to ask the question, "Why is the digestive system suffering?" Possibilities include but are not limited to intake of improper foods, excessive stress, a generalized weakened root source of energy, and excessive worry. A simplified beginning treatment plan to address the elbow pain for this patient is thus: Acupuncture to help alleviate pain and increase blood circulation → structural analysis and treatment from a chiropractor, Rolf structural integration therapist, or licensed medical massage therapist → nutrition guidelines to strengthen the digestive system → life or behavioral health coaching to learn tools to manage stress and worry less.

In my everyday practice, I go from patient to patient with the intention of having an open mind and hearing what the patient has to say. What does the patient believe to be true about his or her health? (After all, the patient does know best.) In essence, doing just that captures the essence of integrative medicine, because from here, the practitioner has an opportunity to meet each patient at the level of that person's being, physically, emotionally, mentally, and spiritually.

DO IT RIGHT, RIGHT NOW

The conventional model of medicine aims to provide quick fixes in response to health care consumers' desires. This has created a snowball effect of inefficient and less effective health care outcomes, which only prolongs illness.

I am reminded of ballet training I received from my master ballet instructor. He touted, "Do it right, right now." What he meant was that if I wanted to soar through the air in a grand jeté or turn multiple pirouettes, I could achieve these goals only by consistent training and perfecting the technical alignment in my body while dancing. In ballet and in health, doing it right and doing it right now yield faster and more efficient results. Trying to cheat and cut corners by skipping the hard work or being impatient with the process only delays the desired goals. Being empowered to achieve health means doing what it takes to maintain it.

EXERCISE: IS IT TIME TO THINK OUTSIDE OF CONVENTIONAL MEDICINE?

Consider the questions in this list and answer them honestly:

- Have you accepted that your health limitations will be with you for the rest of your life?
- Are you limited in achieving your truest potential life due to a physical, mental, or emotional illness?
- Do you have questions about the root cause of your symptom, illness, or disease?
- Do you have questions about understanding your treatment plan?
- Can you imagine feeling more vibrant and energetic in your daily life?
- Do you feel like you cannot move forward in your health until you have a diagnosis?

If you answered yes to any of these questions, then the integrative and collaborative health care approach is important to include in your health care plan.

As with other challenges in life, it is tempting to ignore health challenges and hope they will disappear or get rectified all by themselves. However, our bodies are beautifully designed to provide us with clues to guide us through life as healthy as possible. Instead of hiding your health concerns under the proverbial rug, find help you can trust to face them head on before further illness ensues.

> *"As a result of the collaboration between health care professionals on my healing team and the integration of multiple modalities, my health has been restored."*
> – Jayne R.

CHAPTER 2
The Mind, Body, and Spirit Connection

I have been in practice since 2004. I hold a deep respect for mind, body, and spirit connections and rely on that respect to help promote health and well-being for my patients. My professional experience has shown me that there are mental, emotional, and physical components to all symptom pictures that must be addressed if one is to facilitate full health.

Just as the mind and emotions affect the physical body, so does what is happening in the body directly affect the emotions and the mind. As my work has evolved, I am ever more convinced of the necessity of bringing together multiple modalities to address each aspect of mind, body, and spirit in order to create a synergy of healing for my patients. Indeed, my work as a healer has evolved and feels revolutionary as I help patients to understand that achieving true and sustained health extends beyond the most current and accepted forms of health care. That said, the catch phrase "mind, body, and spirit" has become trendy and is commonly tossed around. Health care clinics, conventional and complementary alike, tout the phrase as the "in" thing, but they may or may not be practicing true mind, body, and spirit medicine.

Before I explain what mind, body, and spirit mean to me as a doctor, let me address the elephant in the room. In the realm of healing, the word "spirit" can strongly repel or attract people. When I refer to spirit, I do not do so with a religious or spiritual connotation but rather as a unique quality that each individual has. You may interpret spirit in whatever way is comfortable; while the definition of the word varies from person to person, spirit's involvement in health and healing remains essentially the same.

For me as a doctor and for the purpose of applying it to health and healing, spirit relates to the concept of living life in accordance with one's own value system and in alignment with one's life passions. In other words, listen to what your intuition tells you about the best method of health care for your specific health concern at a given juncture in time. This also applies to other areas of your life. What makes your ears perk up and induces tail-wagging? What gets you up in the morning? What flows through your body that drives you to live your life in a meaningful way? Some people compare spirit to one's vital force.

When it comes to achieving health, sometimes the phrase "mind, body, and spirit" is meant to grab the attention of the health care consumer who is into seemingly whimsical things. At other times, the phrase is used in a concrete and scientifically driven way. Either way, in general, the phrase suggests that mind, body, and spirit are all aspects to consider when addressing the person as a whole. That's all well and good; however, it also suggests that the mind, body, and spirit are separate from one another, which means using the phrase in this way falls into the reductionist way of thinking to which our health care system has fallen prey. Furthermore, the phrase leaves out other aspects of one's health that are intertwined in mind, body, and spirit, such as mental and emotional health. Addressing the mind, body, and spirit holistically and not as separate from one another is inherent in a true healing process. With that in mind, the phrase could be expanded to include physical, emotional, mental, and spiritual health.

How does this apply to addressing a health care concern? When a patient visits his or her doctor or health care practitioner with a chief complaint, the complaint can usually be categorized as belonging to the physical, emotional, mental, or spiritual realm. However, no matter the categorization, to truly find healing, all involved aspects must be considered and addressed appropriately.

For example, consider an obvious physical complaint such as plantar fasciitis. While it certainly does present as a physical symptom, the true problem will likely involve the digestive system as well as the patient's mental and emotional health. This is because soft tissues like tendons require proper nutrients to heal, and if the patient's digestive system is weak, the patient will not have the proper nutrients available to heal the injury. In addition, emotional strain and mental overexertion are what often creates digestive weakness. This explains why one person's plantar fasciitis will certainly vary from the next, as the background health information of each individual is unique. For that reason, an individualized health plan is required for each and every patient for optimal healing to occur.

TCM PEARL OF WISDOM

Your body wants to be well. Treat it with love, compassion, and respect, and know that your body can heal itself.

SUSAN'S STORY

Susan, sixty-two years old, presented with the chief complaints of heart palpitations, insomnia, and hot flashes. Susan said from the beginning of her first session that she had agreed because she heard I practice "science-based" TCM. "Energy medicine" is considered taboo in Susan's religious belief system.

Over the years, I have developed the skill of meeting patients where they are in terms of their own belief systems. I took Susan's comment as a cue to use words, ideas, and explanations of her symptoms rooted in conventional terms. We fairly quickly got on top of her symptoms by using acupuncture and Chinese herbs, and we developed a rapport of trust.

Susan contacted me again after she had done some traveling overseas, where her symptoms came back with a vengeance. We created a treatment plan similar to the one before, but this time without as much success.

I learned that while Susan was on her trip, a trauma occurred. I told her that this shock to her system might actually have triggered the recurrence of her symptoms, as my medical experience has shown me that experiencing a traumatic experience can do so. At first, Susan denied that the shock of the trauma might be related to her symptoms. I tried to help open her eyes to the concept that indeed our bodies store emotional stress that manifests itself as physical symptoms, often in the "weakest link" of our health chain. For her, the weak link was that her hormone levels were changing because she was perimenopausal. Susan and I had gotten her symptoms to subside, although it would take upward of another year for her to achieve enough balance in her system to resist the symptoms' return.

The process of accepting that emotional trauma could show up physically was particularly challenging for Susan. The process of acknowledging her emotions was entwined with her spiritual beliefs, and those beliefs had instilled a fear in her that any form of "energy" medicine might leave an opening for evil to come into her body. That said, hormonal replacement therapy, beta-blockers, and an anti-anxiety agent, which her conventional Western medical team offered after ruling out cardiovascular disease, did not sit well with her.

For months, we explored more scientifically based therapies such as acupuncture, chiropractic, and even counseling to treat her symptoms of heart palpitations, insomnia, and hot flashes.

While those therapies helped other things, they only mildly addressed her chief complaint. She eventually became so desperate to feel better that she accepted my recommendation to try homeopathy (despite the fact that homeopathy is considered more of an "energy" medicine and is controversial in the conventional medicine world). When guided by a classical homeopath, homeopathy is a perfect therapy to use when emotional or physical symptoms, or both, are caused by a specific traumatic event. Fortunately, the homeopathy treatment Susan received allowed her system to return to its natural state of homeostasis by helping it to mount its own healing response.

Susan's ultimate healing was a testament for her to follow her own internal spiritual guidance system. Her inner guidance led her to pursue a collaborative and integrative approach to resolving her symptoms after she realized that pharmaceuticals would not provide healing for her.

To sum up, mind, body, and spirit are one. Our physical, emotional, mental, and spiritual aspects of health are one. For us to live fully healthy and spirited lives, every aspect of our health must operate in a balanced way. The body is designed to live as a harmoniously functioning system, but sometimes it needs a little guidance. Proper guidance requires thinking about health in this connected way.

> *"In today's world, we have choices for medical treatment that can be controversial and confusing. When I started receiving acupuncture, chiropractic, and body work, I realized that some friends wondered if it was kind of "out there." I found a healing team with whom I was free to question this idea so that I would know that my personal beliefs would be honored. This response on the practitioners' part was supportive. I appreciated it, and it propelled my health forward."*
>
> *–Joy K., teacher*

CHAPTER 3
Traditional Chinese Medicine

Appreciating and experiencing the value of Traditional Chinese Medicine as a medical practice is new for many people who have not experienced it before. As my patient Susan found by accepting that emotions were affecting her physical body, changing one's way of thinking about health can be challenging. I was in the beautiful, lush foothills of Corbett, Oregon, at a retreat to kick off my master's program when I realized I had entered a whole new world of thinking about health.

Some students were demonstrating qigong, a system of body movements that involve breath, meditation, and martial arts training. The students were moving in such a free-flowing and, frankly, completely strange way that I had no idea what I was witnessing. Having grown up with my first passion as a ballerina, the form of movement I was watching was far from the disciplined and strongly regimented rigor of ballet. Ballet is about control, and qigong looked completely unruly.

I was clearly out of my element in this program. From the mountainside, I could see a long way out—miles and miles of wilderness. I looked down the mountain—and wanted to run away. (Luckily, I did not.) The way those students were moving was unfamiliar, and it made me feel a little uncomfortable, but this was only the beginning of stretching my comfort zone.

As it turned out, I was in for three years of feeling uncomfortable. My mind had to stretch to accept the possibility that the world might not be exactly as I had perceived it. Having been immersed in the ideals of conventional medicine thinking in my undergraduate pre-med program, I was challenged to my core with the TCM way of thinking. Gone was the longwinded, complicated, and scientific-sounding language of medical science.

I was being asked to turn my understanding of how the body works from the organized scientific model of atoms and molecules to seemingly obscure concepts of qi ("chee") and yin and yang and to consider pathology in terms of cold, heat, wind, and dampness. There were plenty of times my academic self scoffed at such simplistic and "woo-woo" terminology. But TCM introduced me to an entirely new way of looking at the human body and its relationship to the environment, and I was in for years of inner turmoil to figure it all out. I studied for countless hours to understand this completely different medical paradigm.

To my future patients' benefit, I came to realize that viewing health and the body through the eyes of TCM in conjunction with my pre-med education in the conventional medical scientific model was a huge blessing. Conventional medicine views the body microscopically, and TCM views the body macroscopically.

My passion for practicing a form of medicine that considers the whole person and resists the temptation to treat symptoms and diseases utilizing a cookie-cutter approach only increased. While I respected Western medicine and the gold-standard methods of research common to it, I personally did not want to prescribe pharmaceutical drugs for a living.

It was not until I began to practice that I started to truly believe that TCM works. Over and over again, my patients showed me proof that there are meridians, the channels in the body through which its vital energy flows. I now live and breathe the concepts of qi and yin and yang, forces that are crucial to the body's well-being. Not only did my patients report their chief complaints easing and getting better, they also described the channels of energy I studied but could never see. Western medical science has to see it to believe it, and I am no different. And I did start to see it—in the eyes of my patients as they felt better. I saw it when they stopped limping, achieved a healthy weight, reported their increased energy, and told me of their increased sense of well-being.

BASIC CONCEPTS OF TCM

A cornerstone of TCM is that it provides a framework for designing a treatment strategy to systematically address layers of an illness by identifying physical, mental, and emotional aspects in a way that is unique for each individual patient.

When developing a TCM diagnosis, one of the first steps taken by the TCM practitioner is to find the root imbalance in the system. In other words, the practitioner must identify what initially caused the disease process and why the patient's health was vulnerable to the disease.

In order to understand how TCM provides a framework for the successful practice of collaborative and integrative medicine, it is helpful to understand some basic TCM concepts.

Qi

People who are unfamiliar with qi often think it is some obscure concept touted by people living in la-la land. I once thought so, too. I now see, live, breathe, experience life, and conduct myself as a healer utilizing the concept of qi.

I think of qi, commonly referred to as the "life force," as the power behind every occurrence or happening in life. When a sperm meets an egg, qi is what sparks this union of life. When our bodies begin to take in the next breath, qi allows that process to happen. When we take our last breath, the qi transmutes out of the body.

In TCM, qi is known to travel through meridians, also called channels. The meridians, which are named based on organ systems but do not necessarily coincide with the named organ system function, provide qi to every cell, organ system, and systemic process that occurs in the body. When the qi becomes blocked in a meridian, its inability to reach a particular area of the body causes an imbalance in that system, which, if not corrected, leads to a ripple of imbalances downstream.

TCM provides multiple tools such as acupuncture, Chinese herbs, qi gong, and tuina (therapeutic massage specific to TCM) to reestablish and maintain the free flow of qi through the meridians. Patients who learn ways to balance the qi and keep it moving in the meridians hold the key to long-lasting health.

Blood

In TCM, the concept of blood is similar to that of Western medicine, but it has a more fully encompassing role of nourishing the body mentally and emotionally as well as physically. Blood travels with the qi in the meridians. It is said that blood and qi are mutually dependent, as the qi prevents blood stagnation and the blood nourishes the qi.

True to its foundation, TCM views blood more broadly than does conventional medicine. Conventional medicine breaks blood down to its parts, recognizing red and white blood cells, platelets, nutrients, other proteins, electrolytes, and water. Each of the components is noted for its individual contributions to the body's function, including distributing hormones and carrying oxygen. In TCM, the blood is viewed more simply as that which flows through the vessels to nourish the body. Thus, blood is said to maintain healthy body movement and sensation; aid the mind and mental activities; and provide nutrients for organs, tissues, and meridians, resulting in healthy skin, hair, nails, muscles, and bones.

> ## TCM PEARL OF WISDOM
>
> *The* Huang Di Nei Jing, *a famous Chinese medicine text from the Han dynasty (206 BC–220 AD), says, "Having received sufficient blood, the liver can support healthy eyesight. Having received sufficient blood, feet can walk. Having received sufficient blood, the palm can grasp hold of things. Having received sufficient blood, the fingers can pick up things." This illustrates blood's importance to healthy muscle movement and sensation. If blood is deficient, then dizziness, vertigo, ringing in the ears (tinnitus), or limb weakness can occur. Protect your TCM blood by maintaining healthy digestion and even emotions, and eating foods such as dark green leafy vegetables; beets; eggs; and free-range, hormone-free red meat.*

Blood mainly originates from the nourishment supplied by the foods we eat and what we call "jing." Jing is considered the essence of life associated with the growth and development of the body. First, digested food is turned into food essence by the two chief digestive organs of the stomach and spleen. This essence is then transported upward by the spleen to the lungs, where it turns into blood with the help of the heart and lungs (see fig. 1). Thus, eating a balanced and healthy diet is extremely important because of the role of the digestive organs in the production of qi and blood.

FIGURE 1. THE FORMATION OF BLOOD

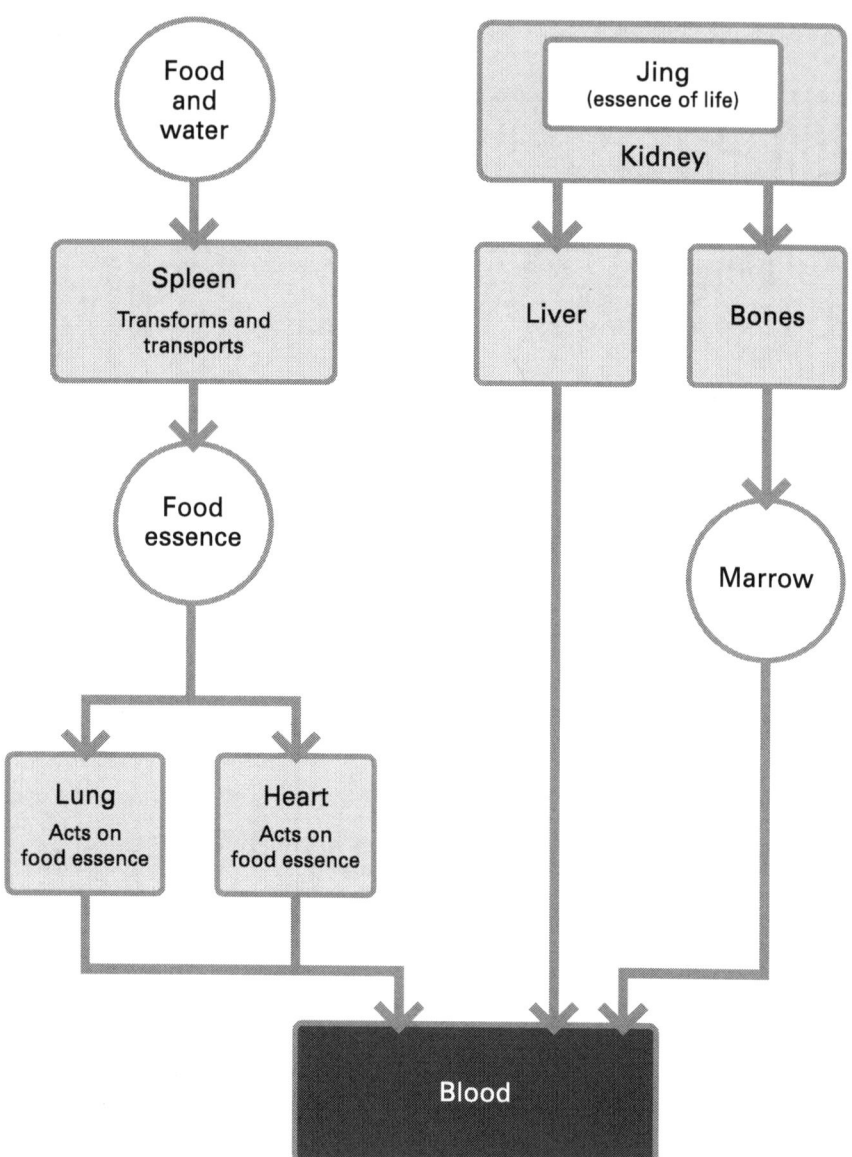

Yin and Yang

In every aspect and consideration of how the body functions, TCM analyzes the yin and yang balance. Yin and yang are opposing and complementary energy forces and are mutually supportive; we cannot have one without the other.

Yin energy is characterized by that which nourishes the body, including nighttime, coolness, body fluids, female energy, receiving, and wintertime. In the body, yin includes blood, synovial fluid, and the body's lipids (fats), among others. Conversely, yang energy is characterized by that which provides functionality, including sunlight, warmth, male energy, giving, productivity, and summertime. In the body, yang includes qi, the energy that makes metabolic processes for life to occur.

The theory of yin and yang is represented well in the yin-yang symbol, in which white represents yang and black represents yin (see fig. 2). The symbol also beautifully depicts how yang feeds yin and yin feeds yang. Without the one, the other will perish.

FIGURE 2: YIN AND YANG

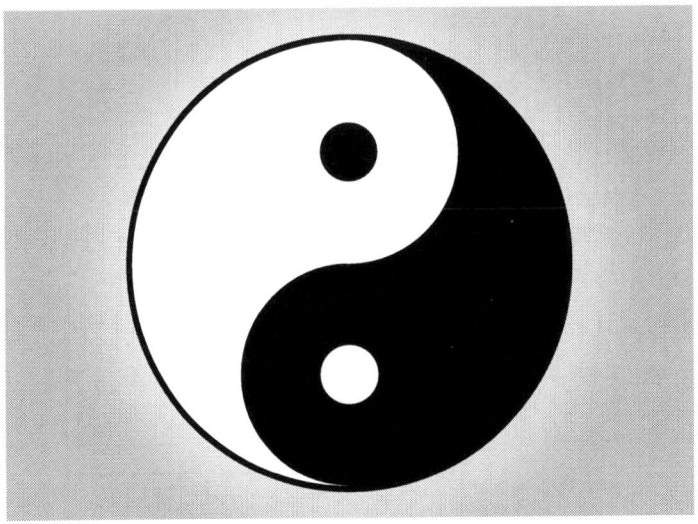

Yin and yang have an important relationship that forms the center of the TCM theory. The two forces represent four important concepts that are helpful to conceptualize when thinking about health:

1. Opposition: All things have two aspects.

2. Interdependence: Yin and yang create each other.

3. Mutual consumption: Yin and yang control each other.

4. Inter-transformation: Yin and yang transform into each other.

These relationships are helpful to remember when considering physiological functions of the body. A primary goal in TCM is to establish harmonious relationships between yin and yang organs (see table 1). Yin organs are thought to have more internal functions and are called interior organs. They play an important role in TCM medical theory and practice, as these organs produce and regulate qi, blood, and body fluids. The yang organs, on the other hand, are believed to have more external functions and are considered exterior organs. The yang organs are mainly responsible for digesting food and transmitting nutrients to the body.

TABLE 1. YIN AND YANG ORGANS

Yin (Interior) Organs	Yang (Exterior) Organs
Liver	Gallbladder
Heart	Small intestine
Spleen	Stomach
Lung	Large intestine
Kidney	Bladder

Though in truth yin and yang are of equal value, as a society that treasures productivity, we tend to value yang energy more than yin energy.

We are quick to embrace activities such as going to work, striving to meet the next deadline, getting the house clean, getting our kids to their activities, and extending a hand to friends and family who are in need. Activities that are more yin in nature, those that act to nourish and rejuvenate, are not given as much importance or value. For example, taking naps, sitting down to eat regular meals, engaging in hobbies that bring joy, meditating, going to bed at a decent hour, and receiving help from others are often considered luxuries we do not believe we can afford. That is a false belief system. As yin and yang energies support one another, it is essential to our health to acknowledge and honor the value of yin energy in our lives. One cannot effectively experience yang without yin, and vice versa.

The irony is that in an effort to supplement our yang energy, we often do more damage than good. When afternoon drowsiness sets in, for example, we may reach for our second, third, or fourth cup of coffee, our favorite candy bar, or an energy drink. These substances create an artificial sense that our yang energy is plentiful, but in actuality, they deplete our yin energy. Consequently, yin and yang both suffer. Furthermore, despite our need for rest, we push forward, demanding that our bodies continue to function. We experience stress coming at us from multiple angles and sometimes worry incessantly, both of which further deplete our energy stores. If this sounds familiar to you, then you may experience anxiety, restlessness, insomnia, endless thinking, and physical symptoms such as heart palpitations and hot flashes as the yin energy of nighttime ensues.

When was the last time you heard yourself or someone else say, "Hey, great job for sleeping in, laying low, eating regular meals, and going to bed when the sun went down today"? In today's ramped-up, fast-paced world, we tend to value productivity and resist rest and rejuvenation. We praise ourselves and others when projects are complete, business is thriving, the house and yard are clean, the kids are stimulated by activities, the Christmas cards are written, the car was taken for a maintenance check, and so on. Unfortunately, we tend to put ourselves down when the to-do list gets left untouched, business is down, the dishes are sitting in the sink, the kids aren't fully scheduled, the Christmas cards are still in the box, and the maintenance light is still haunting us every time we start the car. The reality is, optimal productivity must have equal and opposite times of rest, rejuvenation, and planning. What does this have to do with your health? The answer is everything.

Many long-term chronic diseases can be blamed in large part on what is referred to in TCM as "yin deficiency." Yin-deficient patients have internal dryness (beyond dehydration) that can result in inflammatory conditions that are challenging to control. An explicit example of this process is springtime allergies. If you experience springtime allergies, the time to treat them is in the winter. In the annual cycle, spring is the introduction of yang energy after the most yin time of year, winter. When yin is at appropriate levels internally, the inflammatory nature of allergies is held at bay because the body has enough yin energy to "hold down" the inflammation. Similar circumstances arise for many other complaints, such as autoimmune conditions, chronic musculoskeletal pain, anxiety, insomnia and hormone imbalances.

The concept of yin deficiency is missed by conventional medicine. When the yin is replaced, the body's ability to heal itself is dramatically enhanced. While there are herbs and foods that nourish yin energy, nourishing yin is not as simple and easy as popping a pill. Nourishing yin requires mindfulness in how we spend our energy, in what we eat, and in feeding our spirit.

EXERCISE: YOUR BODY IS CALLING

This simple exercise requires just a small span of time, as little as five minutes. Ask yourself the following questions: What do my body and spirit need right now? Am I hungry? Thirsty? Tired? Bored? Lonely? Does my body need to move?

Once you determine the answers to these questions, you can appropriately cure what ails you. Honor what your body is asking of you. If you are hungry, eat something nourishing. If you are thirsty, drink a nourishing drink. If you are tired, rest. If you are bored, find something to do that feeds your desire for joy. If you are lonely, reach out to a friend or take a walk in the park and say hello to those around you. If your body feels stagnant, exercise. When you listen to the clues your body is giving you and answer your body with the course of action it desires, your health will thank you for it.

Start paying attention to your body and spirit. Seasonally, notice when darkness, the yin of the day, begins earlier in the evening and stays longer in the morning. Darkness insinuates rest. Take advantage of the opportunity the darkness of winter provides for you to rest and rejuvenate so that when the yang of spring and summer encroaches, you have appropriate energy to work and play during the longer daylight hours.

By the time yin deficiency is physiologically affecting the body and causing illness, expect that nourishing the yin will take some time. The path to nourishing yin, and thereby soothing chronic inflammatory processes, is a long and steady one. Reach out to health care professionals who understand this concept and know how to replenish yin in the most effective way possible, utilizing, for example, diet, behavioral health, acupuncture, and herbs.

> **TCM PEARL OF WISDOM**
>
> *Have you noticed that symptoms such as hot flashes, pain, anxiety, and itchy skin get worse at night? It is a false belief that symptoms are worse at night because we are less busy than we are during the day, when we are distracted. These symptoms worsen because they are rooted in yin deficiency. The answer? Nourish yin by eating yin-nourishing foods and valuing rest.*

THE FIVE ELEMENTS

The five elements theory in TCM illustrates how each of the primary five elements in the environment directly corresponds with a specific organ system and emotion. It inextricably ties the physical, emotional, and spiritual aspects of our beings together. Understanding the five elements theory is key to understanding the multiple associations between specific disease processes.

Once you have a basic understanding of these five elements and their specific correlations with each other inside of the body and outside, in the environment, it is possible to hear the wisdom and guidance your body offers. TCM offers an exquisite framework for understanding the complexity of how all of the physiological systems of the body are entwined with one another and with multiple aspects of the environment.

The following is an explanation of various five-element relationships, which will help you to understand this concept more fully.

THE GENERATING AND CONTROLLING CYCLE

The key TCM concept of the generating and controlling cycle is helpful in understanding that organ systems do not operate independently of one another but rather are dependent on one another (see fig. 3). This cycle offers an exquisite framework to understanding how each organ system is represented in nature, how the organs are related to one another, and how these relationships affect our physical health.

FIGURE 3. GENERATING AND CONTROLLING CYCLE

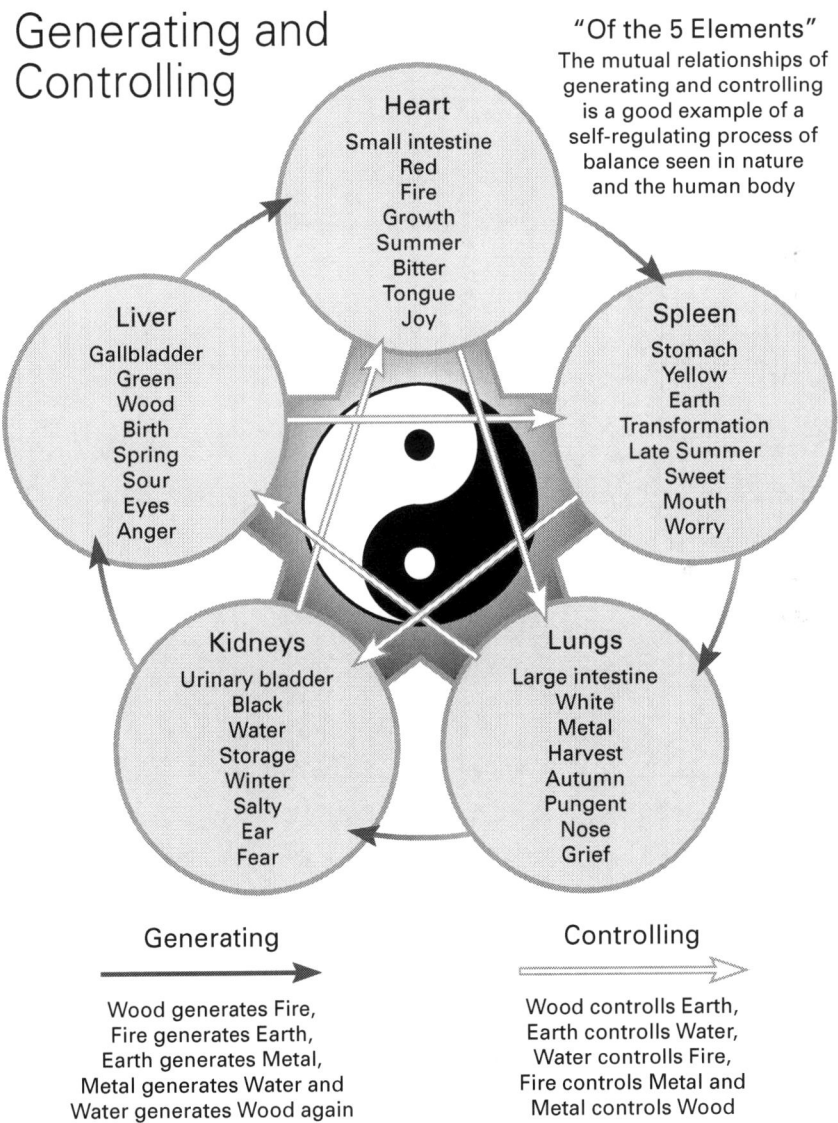

When you understand that these relationships exist and are aware of clues provided by your body, you can be guided through your life in a healthful and meaningful way (see table 2).

TABLE 2. THE FIVE ELEMENTS AND THEIR ASSOCIATIONS

ORGAN	PAIRED ORGAN	COLOR	ELEMENT	FUNCTION IN NATURE	SEASON	FLAVOR	SENSORY ORGAN	EMOTION
Liver	Gallbladder	Green	Wood	Birth	Spring	Sour	Eyes	Anger
Heart	Small intestine	Red	Fire	Growth	Summer	Bitter	Tongue	Joy
Spleen	Stomach	Yellow	Earth	Transformation	Late Summer	Sweet	Mouth	Worry
Lungs	Large intestine	White	Metal	Harvest	Autumn	Pungent	Nose	Grief
Kidneys	Urinary bladder	Black	Water	Storage	Winter	Salty	Ear	Fear

Symbology is frequently used in TCM; this is especially evident when considering organ relationships. For example, in the generating cycle, wood is the mother of fire, fire is the mother of earth, earth is the mother of metal, metal is the mother of water, and water is the mother of wood. When the mother is weak, so is the son. When the son is weak, it drains on the mother. This is seen in the progression of seasons, as spring gives birth to summer, which gives birth to late summer, which gives birth to fall, and so on. The mother-child relationship is used because the mother is seen as a creative and nurturing force.

In the controlling cycle, each organ system ensures balance between the elements and their corresponding organ systems. For example, wood/liver/gallbladder controls earth/spleen/stomach. Here, the father-child symbology is used, as the father is the patriarchal head of the household.

Sometimes, one organ system becomes overly controlling and causes weakness in another organ system it is meant to regulate. At other times, the element/organ system that should be controlled becomes imbalanced and excessive, thereby causing a backup of qi and takes over control of the organ that normally controls it. For example, if wood becomes excessive, then instead of metal/lungs controlling wood/liver, wood can insult metal/lungs. An analogy here would be the child (wood) rebelling and insulting the father (metal/lungs).

Four pathologies between the organ relationships are possible:

- Element in excess overacts on another
- Element in deficiency is insulted by another
- Element in excess drains from mother
- Element in deficiency fails to nourish child
- Each of these pathologies can result in multiple symptoms and disease processes.

PATHOLOGICAL FACTORS

Health imbalances in the body can be differentiated beyond than which is typically given in a Western medicine diagnosis. According to TCM, there are varying aspects of causality, or pathological factors, for any given illness. There are six common pathological factors, which can often combine to complicate disease formation and the resulting treatment plan.

1. Wind is identified as the carrier for pathological factors to penetrate the body. It is marked by sudden changes in the body, such as suddenly falling ill to the common cold or flu. It is also blamed for frenetic movements in the body, such as tremors and seizures.
2. Cold is identified by that which causes tightness, contraction, stagnation, and impaired circulation in the body.

3. Damp is identified by that which causes sluggishness and heaviness. Damp is often a result of a weakened digestive system and occurs from the body's failure to transform moisture. The body's failure to properly regulate the moisture leads to dampness, causing conditions such as arthritis, edema, and feeling thirsty without the desire to drink.

4. Heat is identified by that which "injures" bodily fluids, disturbs the mind, and damages the yin. Heat leads to inflammation.

5. Summer heat is identified by sweltering heat that consumes yin and qi and causes upward disbursement of qi. Summer heat occurs only in the summertime.

6. Dryness is identified by the consumption of bodily fluids, meaning heat dries up the bodily fluids.

These pathological factors often show up in the body in combination with one another. Let's look at, for example, making a differential diagnosis for arthritis. In TCM, arthritis may be a combination of wind/cold/damp or wind/heat/damp. Based on a patient's diagnosis of the pathological factors diagnosed for arthritis, appropriate treatment strategies can be applied to uniquely treat the person.

Natural occurrences in the environment can be mimicked in the human body. For example, those who suffer from tremor, allergies, joint pain that moves from joint to joint, eye or facial tics, sudden spurts of anger, dizziness, or vertigo may experience their symptoms worsen in the springtime. These symptoms are the result of the pathological factor of wind, which is prevalent at that time. As an analogy, consider what wind can do in nature, and then compare that to the human body. Just as wind flutters the leaves of the trees, so too can it cause frequent micro-movements in the body such as tremor and tics. Just as wind can cause an upheaval in the environment, so too can it disrupt equilibrium and cause dizziness and vertigo in people. Just as wind can seem to arise suddenly out of nowhere and scurry from place to place in the environment, so too can it do so in the body, causing joint pain that starts suddenly and moves through the body.

The link between spring wind and physical health occurs largely within the TCM liver organ system. The liver corresponds with the wood element, which is prevalent in the springtime, as trees are generating a new cycle of growth. In both conventional and TCM medical paradigms, if the liver is not functioning properly, it affects many aspects of our health. In TCM, the liver is said to store the blood and rule the soft tissues, such as fascia and tendons. It also ensures the smooth flow of the body's qi and regulates emotions.

Symptoms of wind in the body often have an undercurrent of "liver blood deficiency." In TCM, the liver stores the blood, so when the body is "blood deficient," it becomes susceptible to other symptoms such as soft tissue injuries. In TCM, blood consists of not only the fluid inside the vessels but also any substance that provides nourishment to the body. The liver nourishes the soft tissues of the body with blood. If there is not enough blood, the soft tissues become dry and brittle, like a malnourished tree. If the wind blows through a malnourished tree, the branches are likely to splinter and break. Dryness in the human body limits the flexibility of its connective tissues, leaving tendons, cartilage, and fascia prone to injuries such as plantar fasciitis, tennis elbow, and Achilles tendonitis.

TCM PEARL OF WISDOM

A TCM diagnosis of wind as a pathological factor that led to a common cold will throw Momma's chicken soup recipe to the curb. Chicken is considered to be windy in nature because of the frenetic energy of flapping wings. It is best to avoid all poultry until the cold is cured. This is also the case with tremors.

Another common example of TCM liver pathology is that of "liver qi stagnation." This is caused by chronic emotional stress, unfulfilled desire, chronic pain, and not enough exercise. In general, people do not like feeling stuck and stagnant, so when they are, they commonly experience symptoms such as anger, pain under the ribs, constipation, and headaches.

The lesson here is that a happy liver equals a happy person. Springtime is the perfect time to take extra measures to keep your liver happy. Here are some tips on how to do just that:

- Remove toxic substances from your life that harm the liver, including alcohol, fatty and greasy foods, and unnecessary drug substances.
- Drink hot lemon water upon waking. This drink gently wakes up and cleanses the liver. (If you have allergies or constipation, add a tablespoon of local honey.)
- Exercise moderately.
- Take steps to ensure that your emotional needs are being met.
- Surround yourself with people who align with your values.
- Eat cruciferous vegetables, such as broccoli, cauliflower, Brussels sprouts, and cabbage. These foods have a compound that is known to activate detoxification enzymes.

These TCM theories can cause people new to the concept to shake their heads. I understand, because when I was in my graduate program and first learned of them, I sometimes found myself laughing in disbelief that this method of making diagnoses and treatment plans were part of a viable methodology for health care. Making the jump from studies in cellular metabolism, biochemistry, and molecular genetics to the idea of treating "wind" in the human body was a giant leap, but thankfully,

I have developed the ability to combine the wisdom of Traditional Chinese Medicine with conventional medical wisdom to see our bodies in a whole and complete way.

> *"The mind-body connection is real. My health has improved tremendously by engaging in a multifaceted and collaborative health care approach to health and healing."*
> —Doris C., retired registered nurse

CHAPTER 4
Benefits of Integrative and Collaborative Medicine

For health care practitioners, doing what it takes to provide excellent care to patients is no small undertaking. Each of us comes to a reckoning of sorts of who we want to be to our patients and the extent to which our roles as healers have a place in each patient's care. Do we choose to stick to the rote roles of our professions and treat our patients based only on the clinical nature of our training? Or do we choose to be an integral part of our patients' health processes and be truly present with them at junctures of their health journeys and even for their entire health journeys?

In his book *When Breath Becomes Air,* Dr. Paul Kalanithi poignantly writes of his own journey in exploring his role as a neurosurgeon, first with his patients and then as a patient himself. When Kalanithi found himself on the other side of the doctor-patient relationship, he had to reshape his concept of balancing his skills as a neurosurgeon with the humaneness that was an integral part of his role as a doctor.

Kalanithi writes of how, as a neurosurgeon, he often found himself *right there* with a patient—at the juncture of life and death. He noticed that as he progressed in his training and career, the breadth of his responsibility as a doctor increased. "As my skills increased, so too did my responsibility. Learning to judge whose lives could be saved, whose couldn't be, and whose *shouldn't* be requires an unattainable prognostic ability."*

Unattainable. No matter how skilled he became, the human factor forced him to look deeper than his skill as a neurosurgeon alone. He recognized that he had yet to engage fully with his patients. His moral responsibility to have empathy for his patients was larger than his skill set to offer it was. I find this to be an accurate description of one's calling as a healer. Engaging with patients from a place of empathy is what allows healers to tap in to the healing energy between themselves and their patients. Practitioners choose to operate from this healing spring of energy—or not.

When health care practitioners are called heart and soul to practice the healing arts with compassion and a true interest in their patients achieving wellness, then they can practice in an integrative and collaborative way. Working in this way demands that practitioners do more than what is expected of them when they work only in isolated practice.

As a healer, I intentionally listen to each patient as a unique individual deserving of focused, individualized care. (As a health care consumer, I encourage you to ask for that attention from your health care providers.) I then educate my patients so they understand that each aspect of health is tied together. For example, I explain that not one organ system operates separately from another and that our physical and emotional health is inextricably related. I then work to develop a unique and individualized care plan. No two patients get treated with the same treatment plan because no two patients are alike. My passion is to help patients get better, truly better, on all levels of their being. When patients can join life more fully, enjoy their families, and reach their truest potential, then I, too, feel fulfilled.

---

* Paul Kalanithi, *When Breath Becomes Air*, Random House, 2016.

Complementary Medicine

Complementary medicine comprises a range of medical therapies that fall beyond the scope of conventional Western medicine but may be used alongside it in the treatment of disease and achieving and maintaining health. As such, the term "complementary medicine" implies that a treatment option, which often differs from conventional Western medicine, can complement, or add to, those of other treatment modalities instead of using the treatment option in isolation.*

For practitioners of any health specialty, taking an integrative approach toward a patient's health can be a whole new way of thinking. All health practitioners are trained to think inside their paradigm of study. In general, none of us, whether we are medical doctors, acupuncturists, chiropractors, massage therapists, psychologists, or other skilled specialist, are trained to think outside of our health care boxes when we consider what is in the best interest of our patients to get truly well.

Until our health institutions change the way they teach health, healing, and medicine, it is up to health care consumers to take matters into their own hands and ask pertinent questions of their health care providers. A good place to start is with a basic understanding of what is meant by integrative and collaborative medicine.

Integrative Medicine

The term "integrative medicine" has different connotations, depending on who is using the term and for what purposes. The University of Arizona Center for Integrative Medicine defines integrative medicine as "a healing-oriented medicine that takes account of the whole person, including all aspects of lifestyle, [and] emphasizes the therapeutic

---

* I do not like the term "alternative medicine" because it insinuates that one ("alternative") medical therapy may be used *in place of* another medical therapy (typically Western conventional medicine). I also do not like the term "holistic medicine" because it is overused and can imply that a complementary therapy is not scientific (which is largely untrue, but it is the perception regardless).

relationship between practitioner and patient."* Many Western medicine doctors use the term to denote that psychologists or counselors are available to their patients.

In the world of TCM, integrative medicine means that there is more to offer patients for their health care than most providers offer. Integrative medicine means literally choosing the best of all health care modalities and therapies and uniquely combining them to achieve the totality of health for each individual. In doing so, two main goals are achieved: (1) appropriate therapies are chosen to maintain focus on the mental, emotional, physical, and spiritual aspects of the patient's chief complaint(s), and (2) practicing multiple modalities together enhances the benefits that are separate to each modality of care. The saying "The whole is greater than the sum of its parts" applies very well to the concept of integrative medicine.

A primary principle of integrative medicine is the partnership between patient and practitioner wherein the patient defines specific health goals and the practitioner guides the patient in developing a plan to achieve those goals. This partnership implies that responsibility for achieving health goals rests on the shoulders of both the practitioner and the patient but in different ways. It is always the practitioner's responsibility to impart the best care possible on all patients, yet patients are the ones guiding the course of their health. In this way, patients are more committed to self-exploration and are active participants in achieving their own health goals.

A conventional medicine colleague writes of her experience with integrative medicine as it relates to her practice:

> I believe that integrative medicine is a partnership between the patient and practitioner in the healing process and that it

---

* University of Arizona Center for Integrative Medicine, "What *is* Integrative Medicine?", https://integrativemedicine.arizona.edu/about/definition.html.

combines the best of conventional medicine and alternative therapies. My belief in integrative medicine has helped grow my practice with patients who are motivated to take an active role in their health care. —Kathy Howe, DO

In my clinic, integrative medicine starts with the definitions given here and elevates them to a whole new level. We recognize that combining therapies enhances the benefits of each individual therapy and is in fact the primary reason that integrative medicine is so effective. For example, acupuncture is well known to alleviate pain, and when it is combined with another therapy, such as massage, chiropractic, homeopathy, or a behavioral health technique, pain relief can last longer and be more effective. Integrating various modalities engages the healing potential of each patient in such a way that the whole is greater than the sum of its parts. These modalities include but are not limited to counseling, acupuncture, Chinese herbs, nutrition, chiropractic, functional medicine, massage, homeopathy, naturopathy, nutrition, behavioral health, life coaching, and Western medicine pharmacology and diagnostic tools.

Diagnostic testing, such as blood work and imaging studies, can help practitioners find clues to what is going on to cause a set of symptoms, and pharmaceutical drugs and surgery are sometimes necessary for a patient to return to a desired lifestyle. When that is the case, complementary modalities can help restore health faster. If this approach is not necessary, practitioners from complementary modalities can communicate with allopathic doctors and the patient to construct a health plan appropriate for the patient.

Collaborative Medicine

I have found that when patients integrate the emotional, mental, and physical aspects of their health, they want their health care practitioners to do something that is rare: collaborate.

Practicing collaboratively means that practitioners regularly communicate with each other regarding an individual patient's unique health care needs. They bounce around ideas for the most efficient and effective ways to achieve health goals until a plan is developed. The plan is then presented to the patient for feedback and input.

Collaborative care demands that practitioners and patients alike actively follow the designed plan as a partnership. All parties must recognize that achieving health involves working toward mental, emotional, and physical health together and that each of these areas can be addressed via multiple modalities of care. For example, Chinese medicine may treat depression by first ensuring the patient's digestive system is working as close to optimal as possible. After all, the body cannot make the right hormones if the building blocks for them are not available due to the body's inability to assimilate nutrients properly. Furthermore, the patient many need to be educated on what to eat and, often more importantly, when to eat it, and that they should eat in a calm environment. Of course, if a patient's body is under the siege of stress, eating calmly may seem impossible. Utilizing other treatment methods, such as counseling, biofeedback, and homeopathy to calm the nervous system creates a synergy that works to strengthen the digestive system and optimizing treatment outcomes for depression.

Key Elements to Successful Treatment

Colleague and psychologist Dr. Paula King and I are both pioneers in working in a fully integrated manner in a complementary care practice, and perhaps of greater importance, we are pioneers in articulating what it means and what it takes to create and maintain an integrative medicine clinic. As such, we were honored to speak at a national symposium of mental and emotional health regarding our work combining Traditional Chinese Medicine and psychology in 2017.

Over the years, we have seen our patients get better faster and more profoundly when we work together. When we were analyzing the synergy of our work, we asked our patients to tell us of their personal experiences when they combined acupuncture and TCM with psychology. Through that process, Dr. King and I identified the following key elements to our clinical success with patients:

- The entire healing team has an absolute commitment to providing optimal health care. Achieving ultimate healing requires this commitment, and the pure intention of the healing team drives the successful outcomes for our patients.
- The healing team agrees to mutually and willingly explore possible correlations between emotional and behavioral health and the presenting health of the patient.
- Each member of the healing team has confidence in the others and their respective modalities of care.

Additionally, we found that collaboration between practitioners speeds the healing process because of the following key factors:

1. Patients do not have to retell their entire health stories to each practitioner. Patients typically reveal different aspects of their health to their various practitioners. Collaborating practitioners gain a greater understanding of factors that may contribute to solving a health concern, thereby allowing each practitioner to utilize their respective modalities more efficiently.
2. Two practitioner minds are better than one, and a dozen practitioner minds focused on the goals of their patients is exponentially better than two.

3. Patients feel cared for, which in and of itself shifts their energy from despair and suffering to hope. This shift in energy promotes the healing process.

4. Practitioners feel supported by one another. The pressure some practitioners feel to "do it all" is relieved, which allows each practitioner to operate to the best of his or her strength.

Furthermore, Dr. King and I found that the strong relationship between patients and each of their practitioners is invaluable, as is practitioners having a strong working relationship with each other. Patients feel cared for when practitioners discuss with them their progress in achieving their health goals. Patients do not first mention the skill of a practitioner as the reason for their healing but rather that they felt cared for from the moment they entered the clinic.

THE DOCTOR-PATIENT RELATIONSHIP

The doctor-patient relationship often begins with the support staff that helps health care providers focus on their work as healers. For example, the first person a patient encounters at Healing Horizons is a member of the front desk staff. The staff member welcomes each patient with a warm smile with one goal in mind: that he or she feels welcome and immediately supported. Whether patients are depressed, in acute or chronic pain, or experiencing a poor appetite from chemotherapy, the front desk staff has a genuine interest in facilitating their healing process. Patients feel cared for, which helps them to develop a sense of trust that the health care team will be operating with their best interest in mind. When patients establish this trust, their nervous systems relax, and an opening for healing to occur is created.

Benefits of Integrative and Collaborative Medicine | 53

"From the first time I walked through the doors, I felt like I was an old friend, and I immediately felt better."
—Steve T., air traffic controller

I once found myself in conversation at an airport with a retired pediatrician. She asked me what I did, and I explained that I was learning how to spread my message that integrative medicine, or combining the best of conventional Western medicine with the best of complementary therapies, creates a win-win scenario for patients. When I said "integrative medicine," she looked dubious. I had seen that expression before, so I was not alarmed, though my heart sank as it always does, knowing that this woman simply had not been exposed to quality complementary medicine.

I went on to explain that I am a doctor of acupuncture and Oriental medicine. As I did so, I noticed that her hands trembled from what seemed to be a tremor. She said that her daughter had been strongly encouraging her to get acupuncture, as her daughter praises acupuncture regularly for being calming to the nervous system, among other things. She said she had tried it, but only twice, explaining, "It didn't work."

I did not ask her what her chief complaint was for the visits. (A chief complaint is the primary symptom or illness a patient would like to have addressed. If this woman's chief complaint had been for her tremors, she would likely have needed a series of acupuncture treatments, many more than two, along with Chinese herbs and using food as medicine to see results.) Instead, I asked her how I could spread my message in a nonthreatening way to people like her, who turn a cold shoulder to the idea of integrative medicine. Trembling as she picked up her coffee, she said that she was disgusted that people value science less now than they did in the past. She said she preferred evidence-based medicine.

This woman came from a regimented background. I got it. I got her. After all, when someone has spent more than $200,000 and the majority of one's life immersed in the education, thought processes, and rigors of Western medical science, then opening oneself to other paradigms of care is not easy. Fortunately, there is enough clinical research to support the idea that acupuncture and other complementary therapies actually cause physiological changes in the body.

If this woman were my patient, I would list some of the studies and their clinical results to help her feel more comfortable. For example, studies show that the fascia, the connective tissue that surrounds muscles, ligaments, organs, and other tissues in the body, stretches in response to acupuncture needles being placed under the skin, showing that there are synapses between the cells of the fascia. This suggests that the fascia may be a whole communication system of its own. Also, MRI scans show that the brain lights up in response to needle stimulation, but no studies have been able to determine the how or why.

That said, research is not designed to account for the intricacies of the makeup of each unique, individual patient. As a scientific person, I question the current gold standard of randomized, double-blind research studies for that reason alone.

DORIS'S STORY

Doris has been a patient at Healing Horizons for several years. Her story is a good example of the synergy of patient and practitioners coming together to help the patient realize her true health potential. Doris has, over time, sought care for such things as sinus infections and various aches and pains. This time she came in feeling exhausted and sick, with a weak, scratchy voice that had been unsuccessfully treated by her conventional medical team.

When patients come in after being evaluated and treated by their conventional team, have not yet responded to care, and more sinister diagnoses have been ruled out, I feel a professional freedom to explore that which was likely left unexplored by the conventional care team.

Knowing that the voice is part of the lung organ system in TCM, I asked Doris about any grief she was experiencing, as unresolved grief often shows up as symptoms in the lung organ system. At first, she denied any emotional factors. I treated her with Chinese herbs and acupuncture, which was relatively unsuccessful. I also referred her to our psychologist and homeopath to explore hidden emotional factors because, despite her denial of any relevant emotional stress, my healer's intuition suspected differently. Much to Doris's credit, she eventually took me up on my referrals. It was then that she realized that, indeed, there was grief at the root of her symptoms.

Thanks to her willingness to think outside the box when it came to her health, as well as her resilience and trust to stick to a treatment plan as outlined by her health care team at Healing Horizons, Doris found herself healed and feeling better than ever. She describes her story here.

> I had been ill for a year and a half. After having received multiple diagnoses, gone to multiple specialists, made several trips to the emergency room, taken several courses of antibiotics, and even tried prednisone, I still barely had the energy to drag myself out of bed in the morning. Throughout the various treatments, I only felt worse and worse. My energy and voice essentially disappeared.
>
> I went to Healing Horizons for an acupuncture appointment with Dr. Schulte. She suggested that I see a psychologist for counseling. At first I was resistant, but then I started to think it was possible that a horrendous family situation was contributing to my symptoms.
>
> I told the psychologist I was referred to that I thought I was depressed. I asked her if she thought I needed another doctor to prescribe antidepressants for me. She said I was not

depressed but was grieving over a family situation involving a broken relationship and that antidepressants were not going to help. We talked at length, and it helped tremendously. She recommended that I continue with acupuncture, and both she and Dr. Schulte recommended that I see a homeopathic specialist.

The homeopath performed an extensive intake about my ailments and my family situation. He then gave me three tiny pills, which I took on the spot, and he sent me home with three more. He said I would probably feel worse for a day or two and then feel better. He added, "I don't think you'll need to see me again."

That evening, I took the three tiny pills out, picked them up with my tongue, and swallowed them. The next five days were miserable; I definitely felt worse but stuck with the regimen that the homeopath had prescribed.

The morning of the sixth day, I woke up feeling wonderful. My energy was back, and I felt as if I were awakening from a trance. For the first time in a year and a half, I felt like doing things: painting, gardening, walking, entertaining, and going places. I have felt fine ever since.

Doris's story illustrates the value of taking advantage of treatment options even when it may be challenging to see how one area of the body could be affecting another. Too often, patients shy away from therapies that do not seem to fit in a way that we normally think of when treating a specific disease or illness. Being willing to explore other options quite often pays off in the long run.

> "The mind-body connection is real. The collaborative and integrative approach Dr. Schulte took led to my healing. I appreciate that she and her team worked in tandem with my Western medicine practitioners when appropriate. I took her advice on counseling, acupuncture, massage, chiropractic, homeopathy, herbal supplements, and yoga, and I got my mojo back."
>
> —Doris J., artist

CHAPTER 5

Key Therapies in Integrative and Collaborative Medicine

By now you may be wondering which therapies fit well into the collaborative and integrative model of integrated health solutions. There are many therapies worth considering, and depending on your chief complaints and health goals, some are better to start with than others.

I believe in cherry-picking from the best of what each modality has to offer, from conventional Western medicine to complementary therapies. No two patients have the same combinations of care because no two patients are created equally. Even multiple patients with the same diagnosis would have treatment plans uniquely developed to fit their disease presentation and the varying underlying causes that started the illness in the first place.

In my practice, there are several cornerstone modalities of care to consider with any illness or disorder and to maintain health.

Traditional Chinese Medicine

Traditional Chinese Medicine comprises acupuncture, moxabustion, gua sha, Chinese herbs, tuina (Chinese medical massage), dietary therapies, and lifestyle options. The origins of TCM are lost, as the medicine started before writing was invented; however, writings related to TCM have been traced back more than two thousand years. It is thought that sharp stones were used to stimulate acupuncture points to relieve pain and disease in the Stone Age. There are several theories on how acupuncture came to be.

I believe TCM was born from a series of observations made by a variety of people, that there were combinations of events that eventually led to the complex and thorough system that is the basis for today's TCM theory. Some examples of such events are as follows:

1. When warriors in battle were hit by arrows, they may have noticed the conduction of pain to areas of the body other than the wounded site and spontaneous remission of pain elsewhere.

2. People may have observed that certain areas of the body became tender or discolored when disease was present.

3. After the discovery of fire, people probably experienced pain relief when heat was applied to an affected area. This treatment would have become more specific and targeted as results were noticed.

4. Monks and other people with a developed "sixth sense" may have noticed energy moving in specific areas of their bodies when they applied meditation techniques. Over centuries, these energy movements would have been painstakingly noted, gradually leading to an elaborate channel system.

5. Curious people, perhaps like scientists in today's world, may have started to notice that manipulation of an individual point location on the body could affect many different symptoms. This may have led to treating symptoms that were either close to or far away from the actual point itself, including internal or-

gan pathology. It would have been natural, therefore, to assume that points associated with common symptoms could somehow be related. In other words, people may have noticed that the therapeutic potential extended over a considerable distance within the body. (This has been confirmed by the transmission of needle sensation along specific pathways.)

6. After recognizing that stimulating point locations caused a therapeutic effect, people most likely would have inferred that there was an existence of channels and the flow of qi along them. As locations and therapeutic characteristics of points were gradually discovered, they were named based on the organ systems now familiar to TCM.

Acupuncture

Acupuncture, which is performed by the insertion of sterile, hair-like needles under the skin, is well known to successfully treat pain conditions. What is perhaps not as well known is that it also successfully addresses digestive and endocrine disorders, mental health symptoms, autoimmune diseases, nervous system disorders, sinusitis, lung problems, digestive dysfunction, and other medical issues. TCM considers that pain arises from blocked qi. When qi becomes blocked and stagnant along the meridians, disharmony arises in those meridians. Acupuncture acts to unblock the stagnant energy, thus restoring proper flow of qi and blood and thereby alleviating symptoms and restoring harmony.

Modern research shows that acupuncture increases blood flow and white blood cell production and is effective in treating multiple pain conditions by releasing naturally occurring endorphins. The mechanism of action on *how* acupuncture achieves these physiological changes remains largely unknown.

An excellent research study was performed by Helene Langevin, a medical doctor who trained as an acupuncturist and then became a medical researcher. Langevin's research suggests that acupuncture works by stimulating fascia, the soft tissue that permeates the human body. Fascia surrounds all organs, soft tissues, and nerves, providing ongoing physiological support for the body.

In an article on the fascia network of the body, researchers write, "In the view of TCM, optimal health requires unencumbered flow of energy through the meridians. Of course, TCM does not specify the physical nature of such 'energy.' If the meridians are fascia, as we posit, then that energy may be nerve signals, flow of paracrine signaling molecules, electrical signaling through gap junctions among perineurial cells, distribution of mechanical forces, or some combination of these processes."* In other words, acupuncture may work, at least in part, by eliciting a strong reaction along a meridian where there is an accumulation of nerve endings, capillary vessels, fibroblasts, lymphocytes, and other systems within the fascia.

One of the most surprising qualities about acupuncture is that the treatment experience is usually the opposite of what most people expect when having needles inserted into their bodies, as the needles themselves are hair-like in nature. Most patients describe a feeling of utter relaxation that is unique and unlike any other form of relaxation. This relaxation provides an opportunity for the nervous system to relax so that more efficient healing may occur.

Chinese Herbs

Chinese herbal pharmacology is an important and complex aspect of Traditional Chinese Medicine. TCM herbology is a system of treating multiple illnesses and diseases that varies substantially from Western herbology. In TCM herbology, the herbalist combines several herbs to

---

* Y. Bai, J. Wang, J. Wu, et al., "Review of Evidence Suggesting That the Fascia Network Could Be the Anatomical Basis for Acupoints and Meridians in the Human Body," *Evidence-Based Complementary and Alternative Medicine*, vol. 2011, article ID 260510.

individualize a treatment strategy to match that of the unique TCM diagnosis for each individual, and more than three hundred herbs are commonly used. By contrast, Western herbology tends to match one herb to one symptom, independent of considering the whole person's constitution. The herbal tradition of China is valued scientifically as well as being a fascinating and popular tradition. Scientists working in China and Japan over the last four decades have demonstrated that the herb materials contain active components that can explain many of their claimed actions. Modern drugs, such as medications for asthma and hay fever from Chinese ephedra and hepatitis remedies from schizandra fruits and licorice roots, have been developed from the herbs, and a number of anticancer agents have been developed from trees and shrubs.

The clinical applications of TCM herbology benefit from more than two thousand years of practice and a vast amount of experience. According to Chinese clinical studies, Chinese herbs can greatly increase the effectiveness of modern drug treatments, reduce their side effects, and sometimes replace them completely.

Chinese herbs should be prescribed only by herbalists who have been trained in an accredited TCM school. Most TCM practitioners in the United States practice with a master's-level degree, and titles associated with licensure vary from state to state. Practitioners with a clinical doctorate earn a doctorate in acupuncture and Oriental medicine (DAOM). In 2002, the Oregon College of Oriental Medicine became one of the first schools in the United States approved to offer this clinical doctorate.

> **TCM PEARL OF WISDOM**
>
> *Some of the most promising research in Traditional Chinese Medicine is its use in treating addictions. While acupuncture is known to initiate a deep sense of relaxation, acupuncture performed in the ear has specific indications for treating any form of addiction. The National Acupuncture Detoxification Association (NADA) developed a treatment method known as the NADA protocol, which is being widely applied in addiction treatment centers for the treatment of many common drug addictions as well as for disorders such as post-traumatic stress disorder (PTSD).*
>
> *The NADA protocol involves the insertion of small, sterile, stainless-steel, disposable acupuncture needles at five specific points in the ear. When used together, the needles induce an overall improved sense of well-being. Feelings of increased energy and a deeper sense of relaxation make the withdrawal symptoms from coming out of an addiction less severe. It also prepares the patient for the next step in the detoxification process. The NADA protocol has been studied and documented to show reduced cravings and anxiety levels, improved follow-through in drug treatment programs, and less need for pharmaceutical intervention.*
>
> *The NADA protocol is a useful adjunct in the treatment of any addiction; however, it is not meant to be used alone in any treatment program. Using it in combination with other acupuncture treatments, counseling, meditation, and other techniques yields the best results. NADA has also been shown to be useful in treating extraordinary stress, such as stress exacerbated by the holidays.*

Psychological Care

As humans, we are on a journey, constantly growing, changing, and morphing as life's happenings around us shift. Emotions are the result of chemical changes that cascade through our bodies along with the accompanying physiological changes. With prolonged chemical imbalances, disharmony can show up as anxiety, insomnia, depression, and chronic pain. Eventually, this same process can even lead to a weakened digestive system, compromised immune system, body pain, and nervous system disorders.

The old adage "It's all in your head" is sometimes a roadblock for people given a referral to psychological care. The last thing I want patients to think is that I am suggesting their symptoms are figments of their emotions or minds. Quite the contrary; symptoms are real—always. The important truth to remember is how physical ailments contain elements of mental, emotional, and even spiritual distress. The converse is also true: a person presenting with anxiety or depression will be experiencing some physical complaints, as well.

In the conventional Western medical model, real symptoms that cannot be explained by lab work or an imaging study, or a specific cluster of symptoms that definitively point to one disease diagnosis, often go untouched by a conventional medicine treatment plan. In an honest effort to help their patients, a medical doctor may try a prescription drug or two, often an antidepressant, to see if it alleviates symptoms. Certainly, there are cases in which antidepressants are warranted, and they can, in and of themselves, provide some relief for a patient, thereby reducing the patient's suffering. In most cases, however, it is important to consider other options. The fact that antidepressants are used to treat everything from anxiety and depression to chronic pain is an interesting parallel with TCM; it presumes that in at least one way, conventional Western medicine acknowledges that emotional health is tied to physical health.

It may now be easier to understand why I sometimes recommend psychological services in the form of counseling or life coaching for a patient presenting with physical symptoms. When an illness is present, it is a natural response for the patient to experience emotions such as anxiety, depression, fear, and anger. These emotions serve to get the person's attention, alerting him or her that the body is requesting help. Answering the call of the body by getting appropriate help often shifts the emotions to a more comfortable place.

When distressing emotions remain present despite appropriate therapies to address the illness or pain, the body is sending a signal that there are still other issues present that need to be addressed. Underlying issues include, for example, unresolved past traumas, trouble in personal relationships, and not acting and feeling in alignment with one's passion; these issues may need to be addressed for healing to occur. A good psychologist, counselor, or life coach can help patients learn the tools to make these emotional shifts, thereby changing the chemical cascades that led to their health problems.

Psychologist and life coach Dr. Paula King says that "the mind-body connection is both amazingly simple and extremely complex. Simply, every thought and action produces a corresponding release of neurological and biochemicals that affect all aspects of our physical being. More complex is the science behind exactly how these chemicals relate to any specific disease or health issue. It is important to know about this connection and to make choices about your thoughts, words, and behaviors that support your health rather than diminish it."

Psychological treatments are an avenue toward help because they address the fact that our emotions are the results of our thoughts, both conscious and unconscious. Once a thought causes an emotion, the brain and the body release a cascade of neurological stimuli and chemicals such as hormones. Thus, by addressing our thoughts, we change our emotions and the physiological chemical response.

It is likely that every adult has personal experience with how stress and poor emotional health weaken the body's immune system. It is common to become ill in times of challenging circumstances. I have witnessed faster and more enduring healing happen when treatments combine psychological care with acupuncture and other modalities after illness hits. Acupuncture combined with psychological care creates a synergy that positively affects the entire symptom picture, causing positive physiological shifts in a patient's body.

HeartMath Biofeedback©
HeartMath biofeedback is a system that teaches people to bring their sympathetic (fight-or-flight) and parasympathetic (relaxing) sides of the nervous system into "coherence." Coherence refers to a state of balance between the two nervous systems, the sympathetic and the parasympathetic. When we face life's challenges with a nervous system that is in coherence, our bodies respond to stress in a healthier way, minimizing the chance for disease processes to occur.

I regularly incorporate the skills I have learned through HeartMath biofeedback, especially when I am working. When I am seeing patients, I bring myself into coherence and consciously choose to stay there. I commonly manage the care of several patients at one time, and on top of that, normal business decisions get thrown at me throughout the course of a day. I make it my mission to stay on time with my patients (a patient's time is just as important at the doctor's time). However, it is also my mission to give each and every patient my devoted attention and the best care possible. Sometimes meeting these goals is challenging, but instead of getting flustered, I automatically fall into a state of coherence, a skill that I have been practicing for years now. By doing this, I am able to end my day at work feeling fairly calm, collected, and without feeling overwhelmed.

Patients often respond to my recommendation to seek behavioral health services by claiming, "I do not need to take the time or pay for counseling; I can figure it out on my own." It may or may not be true, but seeking help from an unbiased professional who can help them recognize emotional patterns that are not serving them can help them to heal more quickly and efficiently. By being proactive and getting a more objective perspective on your emotions and behaviors, changes can be made before further illness ensues. Let's face it: diseases are both time-consuming and expensive in and of themselves. Why not accept help from as many angles as possible?

Once patients accept my referral and seek professional behavioral health care, most of them are thrilled with the progress they experience mentally, emotionally, and physically. My patients frequently comment that they had simply taken my word for it when I recommended behavioral health to address their chief complaints. Then, after meeting with a counselor, they can better understand the mental, emotional, and physical connections that pertain to alleviating their symptoms.

Chiropractic

Chiropractic care is a health care discipline that emphasizes the innate power of the body to heal itself. Chiropractic has become more mainstream in recent years, and chiropractors are port-of-entry doctors. While chiropractic is commonly thought to address bone alignment of the spine, it is in reality a practice that focuses on optimizing nervous system function. Chiropractic adjustments are performed either manually or with an instrument called an activator. The adjustments gently remove subluxations (misalignments) in the spine, thereby allowing nerves exiting the spine to transmit impulses freely. The nerves can then properly send messages from the central nervous system to all parts of the body, including organ systems. In other words, chiropractic adjustments allow for proper function to occur naturally and help patients avoid taking unnecessary and potentially dangerous medications that often have numerous side effects.

What may come as a surprise is chiropractic's effectiveness in treating gastroesophageal reflux disease (GERD). Approximately seven million people in the United States have some symptoms of GERD, and the majority of those who suffer think that their stomachs are producing too much acid. They then treat it with over-the-counter or prescription drugs designed to reduce stomach acid. As we get older, we actually produce less stomach acid (called hypochlorhydria), leading to a decreased ability to digest food properly. Then, when we eat, the food is not digested well due to the lack of hydrochloric acid, so instead of continuing down the digestive tract, the food sits in the stomach and putrefies, leading to indigestion or acid reflux.

The actual problem is not having too much stomach acid but that the stomach acid is not staying in the stomach. A round muscle called the lower esophageal sphincter sits at the top of the stomach. Its job is to open when food enters the stomach and close afterward, preventing anything from coming up out of the stomach and into the "food pipe," or esophagus. Sometimes this muscle is not able to close properly because of improper nerve supply. This muscle receives its nerve supply from the nerves exiting the spinal cord and then the spinal column just below the shoulder blades. When a subluxation occurs in this area of the spine, it prevents these nerves from giving the lower esophageal sphincter the proper signals. This prevents the muscle from closing all the way, which allows stomach acid to travel out of the stomach and create heartburn, or acid reflux.

Chiropractic medicine is safe and effective. There are different styles of chiropractic, each with its own niche. Some patients prefer and respond better to manual adjustments, while others prefer a gentler approach. Developing a rapport with your practitioner is important, as it is with any doctor, because you must be able to express what you are and are not comfortable with in terms of style of treatment.

Food as Medicine

Most of us think of food as necessary to our survival because it provides the calories and nutrients necessary for the body to regulate basic functions. While this is certainly a task food performs, our diet has much more potential to serve our health. For thousands of years, TCM has offered a completely different perspective on food: food as medicine. In fact, many illnesses can be treated by simple writing a prescription to eat specific foods to help cure a health imbalance.

To fully grasp the premise of using food as medicine, there are two basic concepts to understand: (1) each food has a specific nature associated with it, and (2) each food has a specific flavor associated with it. Foods are either cool, cold, neutral, warm, or hot in nature, and either sour, bitter, sweet, spicy, or salty in flavor. Each nature and flavor associated with a food can either help cure or worsen a specific disease process. For example, warm- and hot-natured foods can help alleviate symptoms in illnesses that are diagnosed as cold, and vice versa. Furthermore, each flavor has a medicinal effect in the body. For example, the sweet flavor acts to strengthen digestion and moisten the body, while the bitter flavor can alleviate dampness.

Consider the common affliction of arthritis. Western medicine acknowledges many different forms of arthritis, with the most common ones being osteoarthritis and rheumatoid arthritis. According to TCM, arthritis can be differentiated for individual patients based on patterns of pathological factors present. Once the TCM pattern is determined, a treatment plan using food as medicine can be developed. For example, consider a patient with joint pain that generally gets worse when cold, damp weather moves in. This patient would likely be diagnosed with joint pain of the "cold-damp" type. A dietary prescription might be to eat foods that are warming in nature to alleviate cold and foods that are bitter to dry dampness. Conversely, foods that are cold and damp in nature will make cold-damp arthritis worse.

Diagnosing various conditions based on pathological factors and using appropriate foods as medicine is a finely tuned skill; it is best done by practitioners with a master's or doctorate in acupuncture and Oriental medicine training. That said, the following are some examples of using food as medicine that you can start applying to your daily life.

Not all menopausal hot flashes share the same root problem. However, if hot flashes are worse at night and you are heading toward or are in menopause, then do eat slippery foods that moisten the body, such as asparagus, pears, millet grain, and eggs, and cooling foods such as cucumber, aloe vera juice, and watermelon (in season). Do not consume hot-natured foods such as coffee (caffeinated or decaffeinated), alcohol, and spicy food.

For stomach pain, do eat foods that are sweet in flavor, such as white rice and sweet potato. Do not eat cold-natured foods such as raw fruits and vegetables or damp-natured foods such as dairy, alcohol, and sugar.

The common cold can show up in different ways. If chills predominate over fever, do eat vegetable and grain soups. If fever predominates over chills, do eat vegetable juices and fresh fruits. Also include garlic as soon as possible for its antiviral properties. Do not eat poultry (considered to be "wind" in nature), sugar (damp), or coffee (hot). (If a sore throat is involved, this is likely a pattern of "wind-heat.")

When we think about food in this way, then eating a well-balanced diet means thinking about incorporating foods of each nature and flavor into the diet. When we use food as medicine, the need for many over-the-counter medications for common ailments such as joint pain, allergies, acid reflux, and many more become much less necessary.

FOOD CRAVINGS

Most of us are familiar with the scenario of standing in the pantry and staring at options for what we can stuff into our mouths the fastest. And while we may or may not actually be hungry, sometimes nothing really satisfies the craving. Other times, the mind, body, and spirit are immediately drawn to something that catches the eye, and in a flash, we have stuffed our mouths with what is usually either sweet or salty, or both.

Many times, these cravings are telling us that there is something that the body, mind, or spirit needs in order to heal. Learning how to read what your body is telling you is important in helping you to correct an imbalance in your body.

The Sweet Flavor

Sugar cravings are a common complaint I hear from my patients. A century ago, the average person ingested ten pounds of sugar each year. Now the average person eats their body weight in sugar every year. As you read this, you may be hearing the cookie jar calling your name from across the room, and your body instinctively knows what it needs. However, wait before you reach for cookies, cake, or that candy bar you have stashed in a special place that only you know about. It is not *that* kind of sweet-flavored food that will help you feel better.

Most of us are aware that sugar is not good for our teeth or our general health. However, I have found that few folks truly understand why it is not good for us. Sugar is highly addictive because it releases dopamine, which stimulates the reward center of the brain. Liking the feeling of being rewarded, we want more sugar. More sugar consumption leads to something called insulin resistance, which means that the body's ability to appropriately assimilate sugar leads to conditions such as fatty liver disease, cardiovascular disease, high cholesterol, and diabetes. Evidence indicates that excessive intake of sugar also makes us more vulnerable to cancer.

Additionally, sugar intake can lead to an overgrowth of a naturally occurring fungus in the body called candida. Candida overgrowth leads to obscure symptoms such as depression, fatigue, generalized pain, foggy thinking, and acne.

Artificial Sweeteners

After the oversimplified description in the previous section of why sugar is so bad for us, it is hard believe that there could actually be something worse than sugar to ingest—but there is. Masterful deception by the food industry has left the public a confused mess regarding sugar substitutes. Sugar is bad, so sweeteners such as Splenda, Equal, Truvia, and Sweet'N Low are good, right? *Wrong.* I always explain to my patients why artificial sweeteners are harmful to our health. (To my young twins, I much less diplomatically refer to them as poison.)

Artificial sweeteners are derived in a laboratory, rendering them unrecognizable by the human body as something that can be digested well. They also modify our bodies to not be as accepting of real foods, which have the digestible and critical nutrients we need to achieve and maintain strong mental, physical, and emotional health. Even more terrifying are the unknown long-term consequences of ingesting these relatively new chemical compounds. Furthermore, consumers are tricked into believing artificial sweeteners are healthier than sugar. This is simply false. Respectable research studies have shown the following:

- People who drink twenty-one diet drinks a week are twice as likely to become overweight or obese than those who do not drink diet sodas.
- Daily consumption of diet drinks is associated with a 36 percent greater risk of metabolic syndrome (a combination of cardiovascular disease, diabetes, and obesity) and a 67 percent increased risk of type 2 diabetes.
- Artificial sweeteners are extremely addictive in their own right. Laboratory studies using rats have demonstrated that given the choice between cocaine and the artificial sweetener saccharin, most rats chose saccharin.

There is a healthy way to address cravings for sweet food. In TCM, the sweet flavor is associated with the nourishing and nurturing qualities of the earth element, which correlates with the digestive system and relates to nutritional, emotional, and spiritual self-nourishment.

THE TOP THREE REASONS FOR SUGAR CRAVINGS

There are three common reasons a person may have incessant sweet cravings:

1. A weak digestive system: We tend to get confused when we have a desire for sweet flavor, thinking we want "sweet" as in cookies, cupcakes, and candy.

2. Lack of self-care: When we don't nourish our earth element by nourishing our spirits, we crave sugar.

3. Candida yeast overgrowth: While candida is a naturally occurring fungus in the body, it can get out of balance and overgrow when we eat sugary foods and take antibiotics. Yeast depends on sugar for survival, so the candida will beg you to eat more sugar, along with fermented foods such as soy sauce and alcohol, so it doesn't starve to death.

Nature's Sweet Flavors

When the digestive system is compromised, ingesting the sweet flavor in the right form strengthens it. To use the sweet flavor as medicine, eat sweet-flavored foods that act to strengthen digestive function, such as squash, oats, sweet potato, white or brown rice, and quinoa.

When we are emotionally vulnerable, the sweet flavor helps us to feel nourished and comforted, but it is helpful to be mindful of what our cravings are actually trying to tell us. Before mindlessly gulping down a sweet treat, take a minute to assess what you may really want in that moment. Your body may truly be asking for water, rest, something to help you fulfill other desires, or a nature-provided sweet food to balance the digestive system. Then, give your body what it wants, and it will likely release the sugar craving.

When you do choose to enjoy a sugary treat, ameliorate its side effects by combining it with a good source of protein or a naturally occurring fat such as those found in nuts, meats, and eggs. Also, exercising before and after ingesting the sugar will help stabilize your blood sugar.

Coming off sugar and its poisonous substitutes can induce withdrawal side effects similar to coming off other addicting drugs. You may want to seek professional guidance to support you physically and emotionally as you come off what may be a sugar addiction. You may also need support to help reverse the toll sugar has taken on you mentally, emotionally, and physically.

The Salty Flavor

According to TCM, the salty flavor is associated with the water element, which corresponds to the kidney organ system. In TCM, the kidneys do not fully align with the concept of kidneys in Western medicine; rather, the kidneys provide our root source of energy and rule reproduction, bones, and water metabolism.

When we crave salt, it is likely that "kidney qi deficiency" is present in the system, and we have reached some level of exhaustion. We may be experiencing a root-level fatigue, which can be caused by functioning at a hectic pace morning and night, experiencing prolonged fear, and having sex hormone fluctuations. Signs and symptoms of kidney qi deficiency include anxiety, insomnia, hot flashes, dry mucous membranes, problems with urination, swelling of the limbs, and decreased libido.

Salty-flavored foods that serve to nourish the kidney qi include seaweed and good quality sea salt. The high sodium content in processed foods such as salty pretzels and potato chips will not heal the kidney qi, although stress management, simplifying your schedule, eating regularly, and resting well will definitely help.

Other Flavor Cravings

To heal an imbalance in the body, listening to sweet and salty food cravings and adjusting your life accordingly is just the beginning of what to know about using food as medicine. There are three more primary elements with associated organ systems and flavors:

- wood/liver/gall bladder/sour
- fire/heart/small intestine/bitter
- metal/lung/large intestine/spicy

To apply these flavors medicinally, use foods with the associated flavors for clues as to what your body needs for self-healing. For example, for health problems associated with the liver and gallbladder, use sour foods to help heal the organs. Sour foods include vinegar, sauerkraut, lemon, and lime. (For more information regarding using food as medicine, I recommend *Healing with Whole Foods* by Paul Pitchford.)

There are many ways that the food industry could help consumers to make better food choices. For example, instead of tricking the consumer with false advertising by using words such as "natural" and "fat-free" on packaging, food companies could offer real foods, using the fact that they are packed full of nutrients as a selling point. For this to happen, we as consumers must demand the best. Most of us are willing to pay for quality, knowing that the end result will bring us emotional and physical health so we can prosper.

If you would like basic help in making healthier food choices, seek advice from a chiropractor, acupuncturist, naturopath, or natural health nutritionist who honors that real food can be real medicine.

Homeopathy

Homeopathy, commonly misunderstood as a general term for natural medicine, is a complete system of medicine that stands apart from naturopathy, TCM, and other systems of medical care. Developed in 1796 by Samuel Hahnemann, homeopathy is based on the theory that like cures like, meaning that a substance that causes symptoms in healthy people may cure similar symptoms in sick people.

Like many people, I didn't believe in homeopathy until it worked for me. After my twins were born, a big part of my treatment strategy inadvertently ended up including homeopathy. After the twins' birth, I was still exhausted and experiencing a tremendous amount of hair loss, even after having been treated with TCM. During that time, I interviewed homeopath and acupuncturist Joseph Ellerin to join our Healing Horizons team.

During the interview, I took the opportunity to explain my symptoms to him. He gave me a homeopathic remedy, which came in the form of a single small pillule (a tiny spherical pill), to place under my tongue. In just a few days, my hair stopped falling out. It seemed miraculous, but of course, it wasn't a miracle. Using his expertise, Joseph was able to correctly identify the appropriate remedy for my condition. The remedy gave my body the boost it needed to heal itself.

I have now worked intimately with Joseph for a long time. I continue to refer my patients for homeopathy and have seen Joseph's skills heal hundreds of patients. Homeopathy is often the first modality I turn to for my children's health concerns.

Many people do not understand how homeopathy can have such a profound effect on healing. As with many therapies, it is not until we experience change that we believe it works. Sometimes my patients take a leap of faith when I give a referral for homeopathy, and quite often they are glad they did.

Conventional Western Medicine

Homeopathy founder Samuel Hahnemann coined the term "allopathy," which is another name for conventional Western medicine. Hahnemann defined allopathic medicine as medicine that combats disease by using remedies that produce effects in a healthy subject that are different from the effects produced by the disease to be treated. An example is the use of antibiotics to kill pathogens that enter the body.

Conventional Western medicine is a system of medical doctors, doctors of osteopathy, nurses, pharmacists, and therapists who treat symptoms and diseases using methods such as pharmaceutical drugs, surgery, and radiation. Also called biomedicine, conventional Western medicine grew in popularity due to the advent of antibiotics to treat infection. The science behind medications and vaccines took hold, as they saved the lives of many people.

I appreciate the diagnostic aspect of conventional Western medicine. Sometimes, more information is better than less, and imaging studies such as X-ray, MRI scanning, and CT scanning, along with blood work, can provide that information and help guide the patient and the healing team to make an appropriate treatment strategy.

Bodywork and Massage

Many people think of massage as nothing more than a luxury spa treatment when, in fact, massage therapy has multiple applications to keep us healthy. Massage therapy has been and continues to be an integral piece of my own health care plan. A gifted, well-trained, and experienced licensed massage therapist can help discern the type of massage that is best for an individual. Bodywork serves in several important ways to allow us to live our lives to their fullest potentials.

Improved Body Alignment

For my wedding, I wanted to look perfect in my dress and feel like a princess walking down the aisle. After the wedding, as I watched the video of our ceremony, I was surprised to see that as I walked arm in arm with my dad down the aisle, my gait looked awkward, as though one leg belonged to a duck. I sought the help of a massage therapist who specialized in restoring proper musculoskeletal alignment by releasing trigger points in muscles.

I learned that my pelvis was rotated, causing uneven rotation in each hip socket and uneven leg lengths. The same imbalance even contributed to some neck pain I was having at the time. Now, when I notice I am walking with one leg like a duck's, I run to a bodyworker who is capable of releasing the connective tissues and restoring my body's proper alignment.

This style of bodywork is often performed by a Rolf structural integration practitioner. It is helpful for improving sports performance as well as the following complaints:

- stubborn back, hip, and knee pain
- frozen shoulder
- neck pain
- temporomandibular joint pain, or TMJ
- most chronic musculoskeletal pain, a situation in which pain in one part of the body causes another part of the body to compensate, and then another, and so on

Low back pain is typically not simply a structural issue. When we consider the big picture, we might recognize how the interaction of body (structure), mind, emotions, and spirit can have an effect on low back pain. Dr. Schulte and I have found a synergy of treatment effects by combining acupuncture and bodywork therapies. For optimal results, we may also combine other therapies, such as homeopathy, life coaching, behavioral health therapy, and additional bodywork therapies. Regardless of the specific treatment plan, all of the practitioners involved in a patient's treatment monitor the patient's progress and make adjustments as necessary during our regular meetings and through correspondence, which optimizes care for our patients.

—Kirk Apt, Rolf structural integration practitioner

Improved Lymphatic Function
The lymphatic system is a part of the circulatory system and is responsible for carrying toxins out of the body. It also has an important function in maintaining a healthy immune system. Lymphatic massage can be especially helpful for cancer patients, heart disease patients, and pregnant patients. Signs and symptoms of a sluggish lymphatic system are swelling, swollen lymph nodes, fatigue, and foggy thinking.

Lymphatic massage can provide the following:

- relief from chronic sinusitis and allergies
- reduced swelling
- post-surgical recovery
- facilitation of the detoxification process
- pre- and post-natal support
- injury recovery

For a couple of hours after lymphatic massage, patients may experience a runny nose and the need to urinate more because their bodies are detoxing from the massage. This is a good thing, because leaching toxins out of the body is critical to maintaining health. The body stores toxins between cells and around the outsides of critical organs to protect us from the toxins. When this toxic load is not released from the body, the toxins eventually invade these organ systems and cause disease.

Relaxation of the Nervous System
A primary benefit of massage is that it relaxes the nervous system and therefore can be helpful for the following complaints:

- stress management
- insomnia

- fibromyalgia
- anxiety and depression
- high blood pressure
- peripheral neuropathy

Relief from Daily Tension
We continually put our bodies through physical stress, which can result in tension being stored in the tissues of our bodies. This is one of the reasons why we benefit from regular care. As I am writing this, I am noticing my old tendency to slump forward slipping back into play. I can also feel the stress of owning a business residing in my neck and shoulders. Before I was taught by bodyworkers to correct this poor posture, I also had chronic neck and jaw problems.

Our postural habits can literally get stuck in the fascia, the tissue that serves to connect muscles and organs. We rarely recognize these uneven muscle patterns in our bodies until we are in significant pain. Poor postural habits can slowly turn us into statues if not remedied. A good old-fashioned massage will stimulate blood flow and break apart the stuck fascia that holds the body in these painful patterns.

This style of massage can help to prevent injuries and is useful for the following complaints:

- neck and shoulder tension
- lower back pain from poor posture
- plantar fasciitis
- tendonitis

It is a good idea to work with a massage therapist who communicates with your entire team of health care providers, since multiple modalities can facilitate the body's healing process in different ways. For example, acupuncture and massage combined allow for chiropractic care or physical therapy to be more effective, as acupuncture prepares the body to reap the benefits of massage more readily. Prescription painkillers and muscle relaxants can often be avoided, making your medical or orthopedic doctor pleased with the results of your complementary therapies.

Functional Medicine

Functional medicine is a forward-thinking approach to medicine that recognizes the body as one integrated system rather than a collection of independent organs. The Institute of Functional Medicine defines functional medicine as an "individualized, patient-centered, science-based approach . . . that addresses the underlying causes of disease."*

Using this underlying premise, patients have specific blood work or saliva testing done so the health practitioner can take into consideration an individual's genetic, biochemical, and lifestyle factors. This allows the practitioner to develop personalized treatment plans to improve patient outcomes. As with TCM, a functional medicine practitioner differentiates the causes of a disease process and treats the person instead of the disease.

When I sit down with a patient for the first time, my mind immediately starts connecting the dots in the patient's story and symptom picture in order to create a comprehensive treatment. I make the connections between the patient's physical, mental, emotional, and spiritual health and a corresponding treatment strategy that combines multiple therapies.

Recently, when I was addressing a patient's chief complaint of acid reflux, seeing her blood work was quite helpful. It became obvious, from this overweight patient's poor blood fat profile, high blood sugars, low

---

* The Institute for Functional Medicine, "Functional Medicine Determines How and Why Illness Occurs and Restores Health by Addressing the Root Causes of Disease for Each Individual," https://www.ifm.org/functional-medicine/.

good cholesterol, and high bad cholesterol, that she was sicker than I had initially suspected. I helped her to see that we were unlikely to effectively treat the root of her acid reflux unless we fixed the metabolic syndrome first.

This patient's blood work helped her functional medicine practitioner and I alter our treatment plan to include more than the acupuncture, chiropractic, and Chinese herbs I already knew she needed; she also needed supplementation to correct hormonal imbalances. After the patient followed the treatment plan for three months, she retested her blood work, and all of her values had improved. In addition, her acid reflux had decreased by 80 percent.

I have witnessed over and over again that these therapies are excellent for treating some diseases but not others and in one group of patients but not others. Getting to know a patient's history, bodily systems, and state of mind gives clues to which therapists, therapies, and treatment strategies will work best for the patient.

"Health involves so much more than one's body; it is a combination of body, mind, and spirit, which is why a multifaceted, collaborative, and integrative approach is so great. For example, I had chronic sinus infections and was constantly taking antibiotics. My primary care doctor sent me to an allergist, who determined I had sinusitis. Then I started seeing Dr. Schulte, who treated my sinus problems with acupuncture and Chinese herbs. I was also seeing a psychologist, who addressed the stresses that were contributing to the sinus problems. At Dr. Schulte's suggestion, I went back to my primary care doctor, who had my thyroid tested and then prescribed thyroid medicine. Dr. Schulte's insights and her ability to work hand in hand with Western medicine are superb. I am now in the best health of my life."

—John D., IT specialist

CHAPTER 6
Your Emotions and Your Health

I often encounter a roadblock with my patients when we discuss how managing their emotions relates to effectively solving their chief complaint, especially if the complaint is manifested physically. I understand why they resist this connection because I, too, used to live in the paradigm of thinking that my physical pain was physical and my emotional pain was emotional.

The first time I witnessed that this isn't true was when I was used as the model for a needling technique class. My instructor addressed my chronic right groin pain by tapping an acupuncture needle into my psoas muscle (this muscle begins at the bottom of the rib cage and lower spine and travels through the pelvis to attach on the inside thigh). I cried on the table, but not because it hurt (although I admit it didn't feel great). I cried because I experienced an unexpected emotional release, which resulted in my crying off and on the whole rest of that day. The next day, my hip felt better. Since then, I have experienced many healing reactions that involved both physical and emotional responses that led to healing physical and emotional symptoms. It is as if the treatment, whether it is acupuncture, chiropractic, massage, or counseling of some sort, stirs things up to cause disorganization. What I have learned, both as a patient and a healer, is that disorganization occurs so that organization (and therefore healing) can occur.

Emotions tie directly into physical health, yet this correlation can be tough to make for many people. How can physical symptoms be a manifestation of an emotional imbalance? Not only are our emotions related to our physical symptoms, they often are the root cause.

Emotions are a normal part of the human experience, and they serve as a guidance system as we pursue our life's purpose. When our emotions are within a normal range, they do not pose a threat to our physical health. However, when they become overwhelming, uncontrollable, and occur for a prolonged period of time, the emotional intensity can weaken the body and cause disease. Once internal damage has occurred from emotional stress, healing it requires addressing the imbalance mentally, emotionally, and physically.

Emotions and Organ Systems

To help draw connections between emotional health and physical health, it is helpful to recognize the primary emotions that directly correlate with organ systems according to TCM.

ANGER: LIVER/GALLBLADDER

Anger covers a broad range of emotions, including resentment, irritability, frustration, and unfulfilled desire. These emotions can cause the qi of the liver to stagnate, which causes a person to feel "stuck" physically, emotionally, and in life in general. Physical symptoms associated with liver qi stagnation are headaches, dizziness, high blood pressure, and digestive problems.

FEAR: KIDNEY/URINARY BLADDER

When fear becomes chronic and the perceived cause of the fear seems as if it cannot be properly addressed, kidney energy is damaged. The kidneys are the root source of our energy, so a disruption of kidney energy can lead to symptoms such as fatigue, tinnitus, bone marrow problems, skeletal weakness, anxiety, and insomnia.

GRIEF: LUNG/LARGE INTESTINE

Grief as a normal expression of emotion causes a normal physiological response in the lungs of taking deep breaths and ridding the lungs of air with sobs. Unresolved grief weakens the lung qi, interfering with the lung's function of circulating qi throughout the body. This results in lung ailments and a weakened immune system.

JOY: HEART/SMALL INTESTINE

When joy becomes more than a sense of contentment, it can develop into a state of overexcitement and agitation. This often results in "heart fire," resulting in insomnia and palpitations. Because the heart meridian travels to the small intestine, the two organ systems influence each other. Therefore, problems with the small intestine can affect the heart.

WORRY, OVERTHINKING: SPLEEN/STOMACH

The spleen is crucial to digestive function, so worrying and overthinking directly deplete digestive function, causing symptoms such as fatigue, lethargy, poor concentration, and a wide range of gastrointestinal problems, from excess gas and bloating to irritable bowel syndrome. As the digestive system is the center of health, when it is left untreated, a long list of symptoms and illnesses may ensue.

Sometimes emotional imbalances are easily recognized, but they are more often hidden deep within our systems. As humans, we have become very good at burying emotional stress (from daily stress to past trauma) and adapting to make it through each day. For example, when I inquire about stress levels, my patients often report that they don't have any stress or that their stress levels haven't changed since they got sick. Then, a few minutes along in the intake process, they will mention something stress related, anything from experiencing chronic stress due to tumultuous family dynamics to feeling completely overwhelmed in the workplace.

In general, most of us are disconnected from our emotions. We become so used to living from a stressed or emotionally charged place that, as tensions mount, the pressure builds so slowly that we often do not notice the negative impact on our health until we come face to face with a major health crisis.

Emotions and Pain

The nagging pain some people experience on a day-to-day basis often signals that something more is going on than the pain itself. Peripheral nerves send signals to the brain (via the spinal cord), then the brain makes decisions about the course of action to take to protect the body. With chronic pain, the nerve endings continue to send pain signals if tissue damage continues to occur, such as with arthritis or a pinched nerve, and sometimes the nerve endings continue to fire even when the physical stimulus is no longer present.

While this explanation of pain may seem straightforward, pain is complicated by hormones, the nervous system, thought processes, and other factors. For example, emotional stress, poor nutrition, and hormonal imbalances can contribute to and compound pain.

EXERCISE: EMOTIONS AND PAIN

You can isolate how emotions contribute to physical pain by taking a moment to do this exercise. Close your eyes and imagine you just had a passionate argument with someone you are close to. In your mind's eye, walk away from the argument, then step barefooted onto a sharp rock. Imagine how it physically feels, and remember the sensation.

Now imagine you just found out you won the lottery. In your excitement, you start pacing the floor barefooted and step on the same sharp rock. Notice again how stepping on the rock physically feels.

Can you feel a difference in pain levels from stepping on the rock in the two scenarios? Likely, you noticed that stepping on the rock in the second scenario elicited less pain after you found out you won the lottery. The same effect of emotions altering pain occurs with emotional and physical traumas throughout our lives. Furthermore, emotions can be stored in tissues anywhere in the body, leading to chronic pain.

More on Emotions and the Liver

To further demonstrate how emotional health can be unexpectedly connected to physical health, consider the example of the liver and its associated emotions. A common emotion that can show up because of an unhealthy liver is anger.

Have you ever wondered why road rage sometimes escapes you while at other times you turn into the Tasmanian Devil? Or have you ever had the Tasmanian Devil in your rearview mirror giving you a special hand signal while making angry eyes and crazy facial expressions? In TCM, feelings such as depression, irritability, frustration, anger, and Tasmanian Devil-like behavior have liver qi stagnation as the common underlying causative factor.

As we have already seen, the liver is an important organ system to our well-being. In fact, it is said that a happy liver equals a happy person. As a reminder, the liver rules the emotions and ensures that the qi, the energy of the body, is moving smoothly along the meridians. Qi also moves the blood to nourish all organs and tissues. From a conventional medicine perspective, the liver is responsible for detoxifying the blood and is involved with several metabolic processes. When the liver energy is balanced, we feel happy and generally feel well physically.

Emotions of stress, unfulfilled desire, anger, and resentment compromise liver function and can cause liver qi stagnation. Even more, a liver that is physiologically damaged from alcohol or other drug abuse, hepatitis, or other disease processes can cause these emotions to be more readily present. Other causes of liver qi stagnation include being sedentary, being unwilling to make positive changes in life, and being paralyzed with fear.

The body, mind, and spirit do not react well to stagnation. As a comparison, think about how frustrated you can feel when you are stuck in a traffic jam. When I find myself stuck in traffic, just idling in a line of hundreds of other cars also just idling and going nowhere, I feel uneasy, anxious, and irritable. Not only does this lack of flow of transportation cause imbalance in me personally, but people all around the city are also feeling it because they are late to work or unable to get back to their families in a timely manner. A traffic jam causes a ripple effect of imbalance within the whole city system. Similarly, when the body is stuck energetically, there is no forward-moving progress, which can eventually lead to mental, physical, emotional, and spiritual imbalance.

Knowing the signs of liver qi stagnation is helpful, as you can take action steps before the Tasmanian Devil shows up. Potential signs of liver qi stagnation include the following symptoms:

- pain under the ribs (either side)
- headache, especially at the crown of the head
- diarrhea, constipation, and abdominal distention
- frequent sighing
- menstrual irregularities
- unexplained pain
- feeling as if you have to swallow past something in your throat
- feeling unmotivated or moody
- starting to feel short-tempered

The good news is that the liver can take a real beating before it finally gives up. There is also a lot you can do to support your liver and improve its health. The key is to keep the body's energy moving. You can keep your liver happy by applying the following tips:

- Exercise, which pumps the blood and the qi through the body.
- Eat clean foods free of artificial colors, preservatives, artificial sweeteners, excessive sugar, and excessive grease.
- Avoid alcohol.
- Take Chinese herbs prescribed by an expert to move the liver qi and support other body systems accordingly.
- Engage in counseling or life coaching to help achieve goals that are in alignment with your value system.
- Resolve the grip of past traumas with a psychologist or a homeopath, or both.
- Receive acupuncture, which works by moving stagnant energy along the meridians.
- Drink lemon water upon waking as a safe and mild detoxification for the liver.

When I thought of the Tasmanian Devil as a comparison for what liver qi stagnation can look and feel like, I did a Google search and found that the analogy between how a real Tasmanian devil looks and how liver qi stagnation can make one feel is quite appropriate. If you could use a laugh, think of something that makes you feel angry and then look up a picture of a Tasmanian devil. Odds are that you will find it to be an accurate representation of how you feel when you are angry.

No one likes to feel angry, depressed, stuck, and in pain, so take good care of your liver—you deserve it. If we all effectively addressed our liver qi stagnation, the world would be a happier, healthier, and more peaceful place.

TCM PEARL OF WISDOM

Did you know your tongue can tell your TCM practitioner a lot about the state of your health? Ideally, tongues are pink with a thin, white coating called a "tongue coat." Any deviation from this provides specific clues about what may be going on inside your body.

Look at your tongue in the mirror. If you have liver qi stagnation, your tongue is probably purple in color. If the liver qi stagnation has invaded your digestion and caused digestive distress, it is likely your tongue coat is thick and greasy and the tongue itself appears swollen, with teeth marks on it. Does your tongue look anything other than pink with a thin, white tongue coat? If so, I highly encourage you to seek care to find the root of the problem before more serious disease occurs.

Organ Dysfunction and Emotional Imbalances

As you can see, emotions are connected to many if not all of the body's functions and overall health. Not only can emotional imbalances create a physical disharmony, but the situation can be reversed, too: organ dysfunction can cause emotional imbalance. A perfect example is a health condition I recently endured.

Those who know me consider me a highly driven person. When I have a dream to fulfill a goal rooted in something I feel passionate about, I work hard to accomplish my dream. I was therefore understandably surprised when, shortly after starting to write this book, I found myself easily discouraged and unmotivated. I would look at my book outline and doubt my ability to write. I had developed a readership via a column I was writing for the local newspaper and had been receiving regular compliments on my writing, and I knew that many of my readers felt inspired by my words, so why was I suddenly doubting my skills?

I was also experiencing symptoms of fatigue, poor sleep, heart palpitations, irritable bowels, and irritability, and my personality felt altered (I kept saying, "I just don't feel like myself"). Over time, I lost my normal motivation to excel at work and be present with my family. I started doubting my skills as mother, wife, doctor, and business owner. Eventually, I grew to be terribly irritable and too miserable for my family to be around me. Even my daily meditations seemed muted and ineffectual.

My symptoms continued to gain momentum, and yet somehow I was able to go through the motions. I was still going through my normal routine: wake up, check work emails, meditate, exercise, work with my husband to get the kids ready for school, go to work, put my best foot forward as a doctor and team leader, take my children to extracurricular activities, teach my dance class, go home, get kids to bed, and finally collapse on the couch. I did not know how poorly I was really feeling.

After months of feeling unwell, I decided to turn to conventional medicine to get more information about what was happening. I scheduled an appointment for a colonoscopy, which I had been postponing for two years, and an appointment with my OB-GYN. Fortunately, all of the tests came back normal. Still, I was offered medications to address my symptoms, which I politely declined.

I had been receiving sporadic care from my complementary medicine practitioners all along but had not immersed myself in my own care. I finally decided to seek the full care of the amazing team of health care practitioners I had gathered at my clinic. (This goes to show that, by postponing focused professional and self-care when I truly needed it, I am as human as any of my clients.) Eventually, I took my health into my own hands and chose *me*. I turned to a trusted colleague for help.

True to the ideals of functional medicine, a functional medicine practitioner and colleague ordered a series of lab work that extended beyond what my primary care doctor had ordered. Many of my lab values fell within normal range by conventional medicine standards but showed up in an "alert" range in the functional medicine paradigm. In particular, the results showed high bilirubin levels, which is indicative of gallbladder disease. I also had low cholesterol, and my sex and adrenal hormones were out of balance.

Interestingly, by the time my lab results came back, I had developed additional symptoms of pain under my right ribs and had become indecisive and more irritable (all indicative of liver and gallbladder dysfunction). I was also waking up in the night between eleven and one o'clock, which correlates with the gallbladder organ system.

After only a few weeks of following the protocol of supplements recommended by my functional medicine practitioner and receiving the weekly acupuncture, chiropractic, and massage sessions that my colleague had prescribed for me, I started noticing improvements in my symptoms. My pain was diminished, and my bowel movements started to be closer to normal than they had been for the previous two years (ever since my dad had passed). My sleep improved, and my heart palpitations were gone. The pain under my ribs also subsided.

As my physical symptoms subsided, the most striking change in my health was that I started to felt like myself again. I was less angry and irritable. I started to believe in myself again and feel less overwhelmed at the junctures in the day that required me to advocate for myself. Happily, writing this book then flowed out of me quite naturally. I felt such relief to feel like myself again, physically and emotionally.

As with other health crises I have faced in the past, once I began to feel better, I started to have "light-bulb" moments as I made the various connections in my own health picture. Before I engaged in a full spectrum of my own care, I had assumed my symptoms were to be expected, considering the rigor of balancing my home and work schedules. I learned that making assumptions when it comes to my health is dangerous and was reminded that listening to my body's clues is invaluable. Had I not received care when I did, it was likely my gallbladder's health would have continued to decline, making me feel worse and worse and potentially leading to an acute gallbladder attack. Instead, my mental, emotional, and physical health improved enough to allow me to engage in my life more fully again, including completing this book with confidence. This process fascinates me, and it fuels my desire to help others see the connections between emotions and health in their own health picture.

TCM PEARL OF WISDOM

Qi flows in each body organ in two-hour intervals every twenty-four hours. These intervals reflect when each meridian associated with its correlative organ is at its highest point of energy. Do you notice waking consistently at the same time every night? Or perhaps you notice regularly experiencing similar symptoms at the same time each day. Take notice of the time, and correlate it with the graph in figure 4.

FIGURE 4. QI FLOW IN THE ORGANS

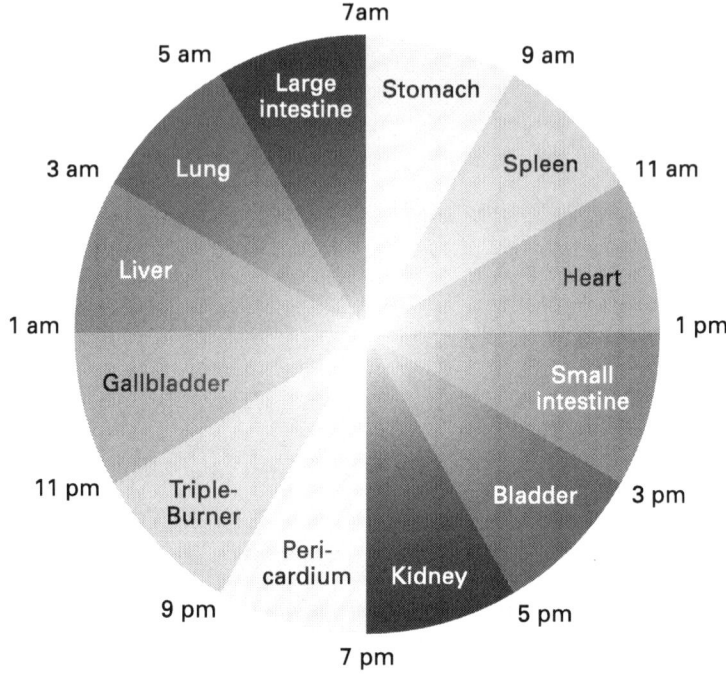

It may take time to start correlating emotions with your physical health. However, by paying attention to your body when you are experiencing both emotional and physical symptoms, you can begin to recognize the connection. Once you are able to do this, your options for getting better will expand, and you will be able to achieve your health in a more timely and efficient manner.

> *"As a caregiver and leader, I am typically the person asking the questions. My personal psychological care sessions have been deeply meaningful and have afforded me the opportunity to be on the receiving end of the questions, especially as they pertain to my own self-care, boundaries, and overall health. In the process, I have been able to refocus my purpose and am beginning to weed out those things that don't align with it so I can offer up my best gifts by being healthier."*
> —Laura C., ordained minister

CHAPTER 7
Climbing Out of a Health Hole

Most of us have probably been at a point when, if we could wave a magic wand to instantly find health and healing, we would. Of course, it is very rare to have spontaneous healing occur, especially for chronic illnesses. Instead, it seems to me that our healing journeys are meant to be a time for growth. Failing health does not happen overnight, nor does healing from chronic illness. This does not mean that the journey is easy.

As a healer, I spend as much time cheerleading my patients forward on their paths as I do tailoring their plans themselves. The majority of the patients I see have chronic health problems that limit their life in some way. It makes me sad when patients come to accept a fate of being ill for the rest of their lives. Often, these same patients feel dependent on pharmaceutical drugs. They are slumped down, tired, and in a painful place I call a "health hole."

I like to show my patients that we do not have to be limited by any diagnosis to live our fullest lives possible. In actuality, we can choose to climb out of a health hole by alleviating symptoms, slowing down disease progression, and in many cases, reversing the disease process.

Illnesses such as chronic fatigue, fibromyalgia, arthritis, and autoimmune diseases such as multiple sclerosis, rheumatoid arthritis, and Hashimoto's thyroiditis are common afflictions. These, along with other seemingly less severe health problems, such as chronic pain, digestive problems, hormonal imbalances, and emotional instability, can last indefinitely. However, through proper and thorough intervention, there is hope to achieve balance and restore health.

A successful intervention occurs when an effort is made by patients and their practitioners to achieve balance in all areas of health, even when a disease seems to be occurring in one aspect alone. When patients are assisted by a caring and dedicated team of health care practitioners to do the work it takes to climb out of a health hole, the chance of success increases significantly.

Being at the bottom of a health hole is not fun, and it can feel overwhelming. However, patients certainly can climb out of the hole and feel healthier, happier, and more energetic. Patients who are experiencing the slippery slope of a health hole can find it helpful to learn to expect the healing process to be just that, a process.

The following is a six-step process to get you out of your health hole:

1. Believe and trust in the possibility of feeling better. This can be quite a challenging step because when you are at the bottom of the hole, the situation may seem hopeless. You may feel utterly exhausted from being in a chronically unwell state. If you cannot muster the strength to climb out yourself, ask and accept help from loved ones. Either way, find the ladder to the top of the hole, and then focus on climbing it.

2. Find a team of practitioners with whom you resonate. Ask for referrals from friends and family. Call and ask to talk with practitioners before making an appointment, or at least meet once with potential practitioners to see if you feel a connection to them and their healing

personality. One way to know if a particular practitioner is right for you is by doing a gut check. Did the practitioner say something or offer advice that induced a sense of trust? Did the practitioner provide at least a glimmer of hope that he or she knows how to help you feel better?

3. Expect that climbing out of a health hole will be a long journey. If you have a chronic condition, there is never a simple way out. Short of spontaneous remission (which I have heard stories of but have never witnessed myself), no one pill, no one practitioner, no one or two or three treatments from any one therapy will make it happen. The reason why a journey lies ahead is because we are created beautifully and masterfully as complex creatures, immersed in a web of emotional, physical, mental, and spiritual connections, all of which depend on each other to function optimally.

4. Recognize that there are layers to your health problems. For example, chronic acid reflux is not just a physical gastrointestinal problem, arthritis is not just a musculoskeletal problem, and anxiety is not just an emotional problem. There is no "just anything" when it comes to our bodies. We have been trained to think of the body in a compartmentalized way, but there are no compartments. Everything is connected and dependent on the health and functioning of everything else.

5. Keep your eye on your health goals, but also appreciate your progress. As human beings, we are good at seeing in our mind's eye where we want to be. While this can be a useful and helpful tool, it can also be discouraging when we are not where we want to be. Sometimes the road to health is so long that we wonder when we will finally arrive at our goal. The process can seem so slow that we may not even realize we have propelled ourselves forward until we take a moment to consider where we started. Acupuncturist, classical homeopath, and colleague Joseph Ellerin likens this concept to stock market. He says, "Know that

the road to health is up and down, but as long as the general trajectory is up, progress is being made." When dips in the road are encountered, take a few deep breaths and remain calm. Dips always occur when we are crawling out of a health hole—always. Just keep your eye on the prize, and utilize the tools you learn from your practitioners.

6. Once you are feeling better, keep things running smoothly by listening to your body and continuing your care. Notice what your body is telling you through emotional and physical symptoms, and then address them in a timely and thorough fashion. Perform regular maintenance checks with your team of providers.

Once we start feeling well, we often become complacent with self-care and receiving treatments, as if we forget what it took to crawl out of the health hole. Health is not something achieved and then naturally maintained without any further effort. Staying well requires regular maintenance care.

Our health is a guidance system to help us live our lives in the fullest way possible. A chronic illness has a tangled web of connections just begging to be untangled. Jump in, accept the challenge, and do it with a team of practitioners willing to serve you by going the extra mile to help you achieve your health goals. I encourage you to appreciate and enjoy the journey as you choose to take charge of your health.

> *"After three heartbreaking miscarriages in a six-month period, I knew I needed to look outside of my comfort zone if I wanted to have my dream number of three children. I met Dr. Schulte through a mutual friend and decided to give acupuncture a try. She was so professional and caring, and she gave me hope when I wasn't sure there was any. I followed Dr. Schulte's care plan, which included homeopathy, counseling, acupuncture, Chinese herbs, and nutritional guidance. I am ecstatic to say I now have the three children I so desired."*
> —Chancey G., mother

CHAPTER 8

Digestion, the Center of Health

Digestive problems are no laughing matter. According to the National Institutes of Health (NIH), gastrointestinal (GI) disease affects an estimated 60 to 70 million Americans annually. The cost spent on these diseases has been estimated at $142 billion a year in direct and indirect costs.

My educated guess is that the NIH is wrong in its estimation of the costs of GI diseases and that the actual cost is much, much more than that. This is because digestive distress can be linked to many symptoms and disease processes outside of the GI system. The digestive system falls prey to over-worry, excessive stress, eating substances that are not really food (i.e., foodstuffs full of additives, food coloring, high fructose corn syrup, hydrogenated oils, and artificial sweeteners, just to name a few). Complications in other organ systems, such as the liver, lungs, and kidneys, also lead to digestive distress. Once the digestion is compromised, the patient is unable to assimilate nutrients properly, leading to a multitude of health problems.

Digestive Distress

According to TCM, the digestive organs correlate with the earth element. Just as the Earth provides sustenance for life on our planet, the digestive system provides sustenance for the entire body, placing it at the center of our entire health picture. Without digestion intact, literally all other bodily functions deteriorate, because we need nutrients to function well.

If you suffer from chronic digestive problems, your body is urging you to take better care of it. If you ignore your body's pleas for help, they become louder and louder by giving you signs and symptoms that worsen over time. Often, these signs and symptoms spread to other organ systems, thereby affecting your emotional and physical states in various ways.

In TCM, the primary digestive organs are the spleen and the stomach. The spleen is responsible for transforming food into nutrients and transporting the nutrients to the rest of the body. In this process, the spleen is the source of cultivating the qi and the blood. The stomach is responsible for receiving the food and ensuring the digestive process continues down the digestive track.

TCM aims to address digestive distress before it becomes diagnosable as diseases such as acid reflux, gallbladder disease, idiopathic stomach pain, irritable bowel syndrome, and ulcerative colitis. When digestive imbalances are corrected, other diseases, such as autoimmune diseases, mental illnesses, hormone imbalances, and chronic pain, can be prevented.

Do you suffer from any form of digestive distress? If so, you likely also suffer from symptoms such as sugar cravings, low energy, and lack of motivation. There can be several reasons why you are suffering, and with some focused care and attention, the symptoms may be alleviated without needing to taking medications or experiencing further illness.

DAMPNESS

One way this concept is illustrated is through a pathological factor called dampness. Dampness is a sluggishness that comes either from eating "damp" foods or being unable to digest food properly. Loosely translated as inflammation, dampness can get lodged in joints and connective tissues, leading to conditions such as arthritis and fibromyalgia. Dampness can also cause low energy and depression. Similarly, when a deficiency is created in the body because of poor assimilation of key nutrients, tissues are not adequately supported, leading to symptoms such as tendonitis and muscle twitches.

One objective way to gauge the health of the digestive system is to look at and analyze the nature of your bowel movements. Now, talking about poop is commonplace in my life. I talk about poop all day at work. The details of a patient's bowel movements can tell me a lot about his or her health and how I can help. At home, my young son makes insidious poop jokes all day long. While my son's jokes are generally limited to making comments such as someone being a poop face, I found these slightly better jokes to share with you:

> Did you know that diarrhea is hereditary?
> It runs in your genes.

> Have you seen that new movie called *Constipated*?
> It's not come out yet.

For those of you who are musically inclined, I found this one:

> Did you hear about the constipated composer?
> He had problems with his last movement.

The nature of one's stool can provide helpful hints to the TCM practitioner. For example, chronically loose stools may be indicative of spleen qi deficiency, while stools that look like rabbit pellets may be indicative of liver qi stagnation.

SEROTONIN

Digestive function is strongly correlated with mental and emotional health. You have likely heard of antidepressants known as SSRIs (selective serotonin reuptake inhibitors). These drugs are believed to allow serotonin, nicknamed the "feel-good" neurotransmitter, to have an increased positive emotional affect in the brain. I say "believed to" because, as with most medications, the exact mechanism of action is unknown. However, approximately 90 percent of the body's serotonin is produced in the digestive tract. Furthermore, serotonin is linked not only to mental disorders but also to diseases such as irritable bowel syndrome, cardiovascular disease, and osteoporosis.

Since serotonin is found in the gastrointestinal tract as well the brain, it is not unreasonable to consider that if you have symptoms such as acid reflux, irritable bowel syndrome, excess gas and bloating, or any other digestive dysfunction, you may also have a mental or emotional disorder, or at the very least be experiencing foggy thinking and lack of motivation.

GUT MICROBES

Another connection between mental health and digestion is the friendly gut microbes that populate the intestinal tract. Science has recently demonstrated that these ever-so-helpful microbes also have the ability to help us feel good, likely by stimulating certain receptors in the brain. Furthermore, these gut microbes also produce their own neurotransmitters: serotonin, dopamine, norepinephrine, and oxytocin. Unfortunately, other substances stimulate those same receptors, too: barbiturates, benzodiazepines, and alcohol.

COMMON UNDERLYING CAUSES OF WEAK DIGESTIVE FUNCTION

To help you understand more deeply what may be harming your digestive health, the following list describes the seven most common and perhaps surprising underlying causes of digestive distress.

1. Consumption of low-nutrition and poor-quality foods. Foods that damage the digestive system's ability to absorb nutrients include genetically modified foods; meats fed with antibiotics and hormones and processed with toxic preservatives; and foods rich in sugar, trans fats, and artificial sweeteners. As the epithelial lining of the gut becomes compromised by eating these toxic substances, problems such as leaky gut syndrome and irritable bowel ensue.

> **TCM PEARL OF WISDOM**
>
> *Excessive intake of foods considered damp (inflammatory), such as sugar; artificial sweeteners; cow's milk; and processed grains, soy, and alcohol, cause the digestive function to become sluggish.*

2. Inability to receive emotionally. The digestive system is unable to digest food if there is an aspect of life a person has trouble "digesting" or if one has the habit of nourishing others more than oneself. Often, it is helpful for patients learn how to be self-loving instead of self-less.

3. Excessive worry. In TCM, all organ systems correlate with specific emotions. The emotions that deplete the digestive system are overthinking and worry. Worrying about that which we cannot change is lost energy, and lost energy translates to creating qi deficiency. Qi deficiency in turn renders the digestive system unable to churn consumed food, causing acid reflux, diarrhea, constipation, and abnormal gas or bloating after eating.

4. Excessive stress. Prolonged, abnormal levels of stress secrete stress hormones, which affect insulin levels, thereby leading to digestive weakness and blood sugar imbalances.

> **TCM PEARL OF WISDOM**
>
> *In TCM, the kidneys are the root source of energy and provide the digestive fire necessary for proper absorption of nutrients. When a person is exhausted, with adrenal fatigue, for example, the fire is out, and the digestion suffers accordingly.*

5. Ingestion of heavy metals, cigarette and other smoke, alcohol, frequent use of antibiotics, and some environmental toxins. Taking in such toxins leads to dampness in the digestive system, disabling its ability to assimilate nutrients properly.

6. Foregoing health maintenance treatments. Consider life coaching, acupuncture, counseling, chiropractic, and massage to keep your nervous system in check, as nerves infiltrate each organ system, including the digestive organs.

7. A compromised mother-daughter relationship. My fourteen years of clinical experience has shown me that the mother-daughter relationship is the most entwined, complicated, beautiful, and rewarding relationship of all. This is reflected directly in the health of both the mother and the daughter. If one is sick, it drains the health of the other. If one is well, it feeds the health of the other. I always say that if mother and daughter are half a world apart, one of them could be suffering emotionally or physically, and the other would feel it in her own body even without knowing of the first one's suffering. This dynamic most

often shows up in the digestive system because this system is about taking in nourishment. This means that diseases such as irritable bowel syndrome, acid reflux, and indigestion may be related to the relationships in the familial female lineage. Studies have shown that mothers and daughters carry each other's cells (not just share genes) in their bodies. Perhaps this is why, for example, your mom is suffering from depression and why you can't seem to cure your tummy problems.

Supporting the Digestive Tract

There are several key ways you can take charge of your digestive tract *now*. The following is a list of actions to help you support this most vital of systems:

- Avoid TCM cold and damp foods that tend to weaken digestive function. These include excessive raw fruits and vegetables, soy, wheat, dairy, sugar, alcohol, and artificial anything.
- Eat foods that support digestive function, such as rice, sweet potato, oats, and squash.
- Find ways to alleviate stress.
- Adopt strategies to worry and ruminate less, such as meditation, prayer, life coaching, counseling, and emotional freedom technique.
- Learn self-care techniques. An excellent self-care book is Cheryl Richardson's *The Art of Extreme Self-Care: Transform Your Life One Month at a Time* (Hay House, 2012).
- Seek care from a qualified acupuncturist or doctor of chiropractic. These two modalities can regulate digestive function by ensuring healthy nerve function from the spinal cord to the organs.
- Take supplements such as prebiotics, probiotics, digestive enzymes, and betaine, but only as advised by a trusted health care practitioner.

Alongside a myriad of over-the-counter and prescription medications to help with symptoms of digestive upset, there are several supplements commonly being marketed to promote digestive health, including L-glutamine, probiotics, and digestive enzymes. While each of these substances may or may not have a valuable place in treating some digestive imbalances, they are unlikely to get to the root of a digestive problem if the previous list of factors are not considered and addressed appropriately. Even if one or more of these substances provides some relief, the root of the digestive problem will likely remain present. When seeking care from a health care professional, it is more efficient in the long run to find someone who can make the connects between each system of the body, emotionally and physically.

A pill will not solve your problems. It is not a stretch to relate the quality of our food and our emotions to our physical health, even when considered purely from a Western medical perspective. When you take the time to address your symptoms properly by adjusting your lifestyle and looking deeper at possible factors affecting your digestion, you will be able to avoid side effects associated with medications as well as costly health ramifications in the future.

> *"I had been seeing Dr. Schulte for a while to treat migraine headaches. My struggle with them had increased, and she said that we needed to "address my digestive system." I wasn't sure what she meant, but I trusted her judgment. The course of treatment that she recommended included tests for food sensitivities along with acupuncture, chiropractic, and massage therapies. After I made changes in my diet and exercise and had done the combination of treatments, it became clear that food was at the center of the migraines. Now I know about how imbalances in digestion can stress my other systems and my overall well-being.*
> *I am so grateful for every pain-free day."*
> —Peggy S., teacher

CHAPTER 9
Finding the Delicate Balance to Achieving Optimal Health

Occasionally, when I mention potential causative factors such as food sensitivities and stress to a patient's disease process, the patient replies with something like, "I didn't used to be sensitive to that food," or "I'm not under any more stress than usual." What patients tend not to realize is that it may take a while for a food sensitivity, stress, or some other insult to the system to manifest as symptoms. To explain why emotional, physical, and spiritual stressors can tip us into a disease state at one time in our lives but not at others, I use the analogy of a teeter-totter.

Imagine you are sitting on one end of a teeter-totter and the other end is where stressors pile up one at a time. You start out in balance, but as the stressors increase on the other end, you go higher and higher into the air, and if the stressors become too overwhelming for you to stay upright on the teeter-totter, you will topple over into a "dis-ease" state of being. While your body gives you clues that your system is becoming less and less stable as you rise on the teeter-totter, you may not notice that your system is in trouble until one too many stressors cause you to tip over into the "dis-ease" state.

The Teeter-Totter: A Case Study

Consider a thirty-three-year-old female patient with the chief complaint of menstrual cramps. The patient reported that her cramps began seven months after she gave birth to her third child. After I collected her complete health history, I learned that she had a history of a dairy sensitivity and that the family pet had passed away six months after the birth. The patient also described chronic tendonitis in her left elbow, neck pain, and fatigue. After I examined her, I explained that from a TCM perspective, she had "blood deficiency leading to blood stagnation with cold in the uterus," which was causing her menstrual cramps.

When she asked me what caused this, I explained that going through a third pregnancy and childbirth and the general stress of raising children were likely the primary contributors. She reasoned that if this were the case, she would have had menstrual cramps long before then, as she had already been a mother for several years. I then explained the teeter-totter phenomenon to her. Without realizing it, she was teetering on tottering into a "dis-ease" state even before her child was born. After childbirth, she was closer than ever to tipping over, and the loss of the family pet was the event that pushed her over.

When we discussed the pet's death further, she admitted it had been hard dealing with her own grief while also worrying about that of her children. This was when my diagnosis seemed even more on point. I explained that in TCM, the emotion of worry depletes digestive function, which leads to blood deficiency. Furthermore, she and her family had developed a habit of having ice cream in the evenings. I explained that the cold, damp quality of the ice cream was also contributing to her cramps. We discussed that when she was stronger and under less stress, the dairy would be less likely to cause problems for her.

Understanding this dynamic can be helpful in learning how to make yourself more secure on your end of the teeter-totter. While we can make our bodies less likely to tip over into a disease process by eliminating some stressors, we have much more power to increase the weight and security on our end of the teeter-totter, to continue the analogy. When we make sure our bodies are balanced and well nourished, we gain strength and power, thus preventing the stressors, which often cannot be avoided, from piling up and tipping us over into illness.

The Pottery Analogy

I think of the collaborative and integrative approach to health to be analogous to the art of making pottery. (If you are not a potter but you saw the movie *Ghost*, you probably know how a potter works and will be able to appreciate my point. If you didn't see it, put it on your to-watch list!) Our general health can be likened to clay on a potter's wheel being shaped into a vase; the clay being shaped is our health, and the hands on the clay and the wheel itself are guiding forces, or influences, on our health.

To shape a beautifully symmetrical vase on a spinning potter's wheel, the potter recognizes that each particle of clay is dependent on the integrity and balance of the clay throughout the entire piece. Should part of the clay become weak or subjected to outside forces that disrupt the integrity, the whole vase becomes weakened and vulnerable and, if not corrected, will just fold over and collapse.

At the beginning of the famous pottery scene in *Ghost*, Molly, played by Demi Moore, is sculpting a symmetrical vase on her potter's wheel. She moves her hands on the spinning clay, using disciplined and even pressure as she sculpts the vase. When Sam, played by the phenomenally talented Patrick Swayze, enters the room (with his shirt off, thank you very much), Molly becomes distracted (and understandably so). Newton's third law of physics, which states that for every action there is an equal and opposite reaction, now comes into play. Molly's once-steady hands begin to apply pressure to the vase unevenly, causing the spinning vase to become unbalanced and wobbly.

Our health, like the clay in Molly's talented hands, can be strong enough to withstand many firings in the kiln of regular stress. But when it is placed under too much pressure, without correction, our health can collapse, just as unbalanced pressure will collapse a clay vase.

The Sphere of Health

Imagine that we all enter the world as a perfect sphere of health. (Of course, in actuality, none of us enters the world perfectly healthy.) A goal we all aspire to is to maintain all aspects of that near-perfect sphere of health—physical, mental, emotional, and spiritual—so that we can live the most fulfilling lives possible. To function properly, every cell, organ, nerve, meridian of energy, artery, vein, joint, endocrine (hormone) gland, hormone, neurotransmitter, thought, and emotion is connected to and dependent on the others. Considering Newton's third law, it stands to reason that should any one of these body parts become compromised in any way and for any reason (physical, mental, emotional, or spiritual), there will be an equal and opposite reaction somewhere else in the system.

Let's apply this concept to a relatively healthy adult we will call Rick. Rick is a husband and father and has a job he loves. Overall, he feels good, has good energy and a healthy attitude toward life, and is able to participate in golf, his favorite hobby. One day, Rick strains his back at work. Considering that every action has an equal and opposite reaction in his system, his back strain almost immediately wreaks havoc in other parts of his musculoskeletal system. Rick's once-balanced sphere of health is now a wobbly, slightly flattened obloid. His pain eases some, although his physical body is now imbalanced. Still, his system compensates, which allows him to continue to function fairly well for some time. (He does notice that his golf game is off, but he does not know why).

Three weeks after Rick's injury, his sister, whom he is quite attached to, rapidly becomes ill and passes away. Rick is grief-stricken, but feeling like he must be the strong one in the family, he stuffs his feelings. This unexpressed emotion produces an equal and opposite reaction in his lungs and immune system. (Remember that the lungs, immune system, and grief are connected in TCM.)

Now having compromised lungs, Rick becomes more vulnerable to diseases associated with the lung organ system, such as allergies, bronchitis, skin conditions, and pneumonia. Sure enough, he eventually catches a cold and is unable to recover as quickly as he would have just two months before. Rick's "sphere" of health, now a squashed obloid, is even more wobbly, and functioning well physically, emotionally, and mentally has become even more challenging for him.

Subconsciously, to cope with his stuffed grief and nagging body aches, Rick turns to alcohol, chips, and candy bars for comfort. This, of course, negatively impacts his digestive system and leads to blood sugar imbalances, high blood pressure, and high cholesterol. His back pain heightens. At his annual physical, his blood workup shows elevated glucose and cholesterol. The doctor prescribes both a statin and a blood pressure medication. While he's at it, Rick asks his doctor for some painkillers for his back. Unbeknownst to him, these medications cause side effects that produce yet more equal and opposite reactions. Rick's sphere of health is now a smashed blob as he collapses into a folded heap of clay on his potter's wheel of life.

RESTORING THE SPHERE OF HEALTH

The good news for Rick is that he can rebuild and reshape his health into a smooth, round, glowing sphere once again when he decides to take back his health. He doesn't know where to start, so he takes the advice of a friend who recommends a chiropractor and massage therapist for his body aches and pains. The treatments restore his musculoskeletal alignment, but he still has some other symptoms and accepts a referral to an acupuncturist.

The acupuncture helps to resolve Rick's pain and boost his energy. The acupuncturist also helps him realize that he has unresolved grief from the loss of his sister and refers him to a homeopath and psychologist to address his grief. The homeopathy remedy eases his emotional pain, so he is able to make healthier food choices, thereby improving his digestion and strengthening his immune system. His blood sugar, blood pressure, and cholesterol stabilize, and he is able to stop his medications. Finally, Rick feels well-rounded in his health again and is able to partake in his life's activities more fully. He has restored his sphere of health.

The Healing Horizons Wellness Accumulation Program

My team and I developed the Healing Horizons Wellness Accumulation Program with stories like Rick's in mind. We combined our wealth of knowledge and years of experience with our desire to create the most effective health care strategy possible to help patients reach their truest potential in living a healthy and vibrant life.

The program is designed to be taken over the course of three months, during which the patient receives two or three treatments a week. It is designed for patients who are willing to commit and invest time, energy, and money into their healing process. It is for those who are willing to roll up their shirtsleeves, get involved in their health care, and stand at the helm of creating health and wellness for themselves.

The results of the program have been sensational. The synergy created by patients and their team of practitioners as they work together to achieve health goals set forth by the patients themselves is phenomenal. I believe the success of the program is driven by the fact that the intentions and goals of the practitioners match those of the patients. This, combined with the synergy of clinical outcomes that occur when therapies are used together, had led to the healing and well-being of participating patients. The therapies chosen for the program are uniquely designed by each patient's health coach to accommodate the patient's specific care needs.

Our practitioners regularly meet face-to-face to discuss each patient's progress. During these meetings, ideas arise that help the practitioners tailor treatment plans to suit each individual patient. During this collaboration, practitioners share specific aspects of a particular patient's health picture with the other practitioners. This information can help that practitioner tailor his or her treatment approach.

For example, consider a patient with chronic lower back pain whose goal is to recover from the pain in order to live a fuller life. I differentiated the pain symptom and determined that the patient is suffering from a root-level fatigue, leaving the back unable to heal. Meanwhile, the chiropractor has noticed subluxations in the spine and brings this up at the meeting. When the chiropractor reports that there is a misalignment at a specific vertebral level, I am able to apply this information to the treatment plan for the patient by incorporating acupuncture points to relieve the soft tissue tension pulling on the vertebra. Now, in the acupuncture treatment protocol for this patient, I can address the root-level fatigue and facilitate the healing at the vertebra. My treatment approach with the patient will be more powerful with the information from the chiropractor than without it.

Jennifer B., who participated in the Wellness Accumulation Plan, compared the value of the three-month plan to paying for an MRI. During her program, Jennifer corrected her high blood sugar, lost weight, greatly reduced chronic back and knee pain, began addressing her anxiety, and regulated her menstrual cycle. By being proactive and using collaborative and integrative care in a preventive way, Jennifer ultimately achieved her health goals for "the cost of an MRI." She also saw so much value from her first program that she went on to do a second one to get to the root of her chronic anxiety. In doing so, she reduced her overall health care costs by reducing the number of medications she needed and avoiding costly medical testing and procedures.

Investing in your health now by using a truly collaborative and integrated health care approach can reduce future health costs for you, too. When more health care consumers demand and expect this level of care, I believe the health care industry will respond appropriately.

"The collaborative and integrative care I have received from Dr. Schulte and her team has changed my life. I never thought I would get to where I am today. They helped me understand my mind-body connection."
—Jennifer B., mother, political activist

CHAPTER 10

Snapshots of Integrated Health Solutions

Addressing the specific conditions of anxiety, depression, and musculoskeletal pain are good examples of how an integrated approach to health care can make the difference between poor health and a vibrant life. The following are examples of how that integrated approach may be applied.

Anxiety

Human emotions are meant to serve as a guidance system through life, similar to a GPS system in a car. Your body provides clues via emotions to guide you toward a fulfilling, safe, and healthy life. If you suffer from anxiety, depression, or both, you can use these emotional cues to resolve their root causes with the help of a team of integrative health practitioners.

Anxiety is prevalent in today's high-paced, high-stress environment. People who have anxiety may experience heart palpitations, incessant worry, and general restlessness and agitation. The anxiety may come from a known root cause such as an impending job loss or having a sick loved one. However, anxiety may also feel "unrooted" in that the cause is unknown. For anxiety of both kinds, patients are commonly prescribed antianxiety medication, which is often a huge disadvantage for them.

MEDICATIONS

When medications are used to cover symptoms of anxiety, the opportunity to explore what can be changed to achieve personal control of health diminishes. Appropriate questions to ask yourself if you experience anxiety include those found in this list:

- Am I headed in a direction that aligns with my life's purpose?
- Am I living in accordance with my value system?
- Is my body asking me to pay attention to an imbalance in my health?
- Do I believe I deserve to be nourished physically, emotionally, and spiritually?

"FIRE" IN THE BODY

Anxiety in the body can be compared to a wildfire in nature. While a wildfire can be started by something as obvious as an explosive lightning strike, one may also be ignited by a minute spark of electricity. The degree to which the fire burns is related to the conditions on the ground. The more well-nourished and moist the ground, the less potential there is for the fire to run rampant.

Much like a fire, anxiety in the body presents as heat rising, resulting in frenetic energy going upward and outward in the body. The physiological results may include insomnia, heart palpitations, hot flushes, upset stomach, and trembling, among others. The key to treating anxiety at its root is to find ways to anchor the unsettled energy by nourishing your physiological landscape. One of the best ways to change your body's landscape is by nourishing it mentally, emotionally, and physically.

EXPERIENTIAL THERAPIES

Psychologist and life coach Dr. Paula King has been clinically addressing the facets of anxiety her whole career. Having worked collaboratively with the practitioners at Healing Horizons Integrated Health Solutions for many years, Dr. King observes that "anxiety is a core issue for nearly every patient we see in our clinic." By combining her work with complementary modalities, her patients receive much quicker and more efficacious results. She finds cognitive behavioral therapy (CBT), a type of psychotherapy in which negative thoughts are challenged to establish healthier behavior and treat mood disorders, to be very helpful. Dr. King also employs a myriad of other tools, such emotional freedom technique (EFT) and eye movement desensitization and reprocessing (EMDR), to foster a change in the physiological response to stress, often resulting in more immediate results. EFT, also called "tapping," is a unique treatment that combines acupuncture-point theory with psychological intervention to calm the nervous system in response to a specific emotional response. EMDR modulates the nervous system response by desensitizing the response when recalling a trauma.

Acupuncture and other therapies in TCM can also reduce anxiety symptoms. Stress hormones that are out of balance, particularly from living in fight-or-flight mode for extended periods of time, are commonly the root cause of anxiety. Researchers at Georgetown University showed that acupuncture reduces the body's production of stress hormones, inducing a state of relaxation.

FOOD AS MEDICINE

As with many conditions, food can be used to nourish the body to make it less vulnerable to anxiety. Hot-natured foods such as coffee (caffeinated or decaffeinated) and alcohol heighten anxiety levels, as consuming them is like adding gasoline to a fire. Conversely, foods that moisten and nourish the body serve to cool it and draw frenetic energy downward. Foods that are especially cool and slippery in nature include eggs, pears, and asparagus.

BODYWORK

Massage and other forms of bodywork are excellent ways to calm the nervous system and address anxiety. Bodywork techniques such as medical message, craniosacral therapy, and reflexology can help you tune in to your physical body and step away from the stress that causes your mind to race. As you work together with your bodyworker to release the tension in your muscles, mental tension in your mind will follow suit, resulting in an efficiently operating mind-body connection. It is in this calm and relaxed space that healing occurs.

Once you are in a state of anxiety, navigating a plan back to health can be overwhelming. It is important to find a team of health care practitioners who are willing to hear your goals and think outside of the pharmaceutical box to help you reestablish balanced emotional and physical health. Remember that medications do not heal; they may help reduce specific symptoms but are also likely to cause side effects.

ANXIETY AND VISUALIZING YOUR DAY

One of my favorite ways to combat anxiety for myself is to take quiet time each morning to "create my day." I learned this technique in the sixth grade, when I auditioned to sit in first chair. I would practice my flute solo in my head three times. If I messed up in my mind's eye, I would start over. Once I got it perfect three times, I felt ready to win first chair—which I did.

Here is a guided meditation exercise you can use to allow yourself to feel calm, cool, and collected.

EXERCISE: "CREATE YOUR DAY" MEDITATION

Find a place in your home that feels especially sacred to you. Sit comfortably. Close your eyes and take a few cleansing breaths. Feel connected to your center or to your breath. Shift your thinking to give thanks to that for which you are grateful. Imagine the day's coming events in your mind's eye. See yourself moving through your day, acting with love and kindness toward everyone you meet in your path. Image yourself conducting tasks calmly. Create the day that you want to have. Once you feel at peace with the day you have created in your mind, give thanks again to the powers that be, and gently open your eyes.

Depression

Patients often experience depression along with anxiety, although they can experience either one independent of the other. Depression is a mood disorder with symptoms that vary widely. Most commonly, symptoms of depression include feelings of sadness, loss of interest or pleasure in activities once enjoyed, changes in appetite and sleep patterns, fatigue, feelings of worthlessness and guilt, foggy thinking, and thoughts of death or suicide. Depression can also result from a sense of unfulfilled desire or from a need not being met. When the body's energy is not flowing properly, as in the presence of chronic pain, depression often follows.

In the current allopathic model, a person suffering from depression is often prescribed an antidepressant. In fact, according the Centers for Disease Control and Prevention, antidepressants are the most commonly prescribed drug in the United States. In my experience, antidepressants are among the most common *unnecessarily prescribed* drugs to treat both depression and chronic pain.

A CASE STUDY OF DEPRESSION

Denise is a forty-nine-year-old woman who presented with the chief complaint of depression. She was prescribed an antidepressant by her convention Western medical doctor. Even if her depression had lessened in severity, she was likely to experience a myriad of unwanted side effects, ranging from weight gain and loss of libido to nausea and constipation.

Denise's complete health history showed that she also had the following health issues:

- irritable bowel syndrome
- acid reflux
- excess gas or bloating after eating
- fatigue
- joint pain
- aching muscles
- excessive worry
- foggy thinking

Current research shows that microbial gut species are linked to emotional and mental health, and with Denise's cluster of symptoms, it was likely that her depression was related to poor digestive health. Her health care team developed the following effective approach to her chief complaint of depression:

- Restore a proper balance of gut microbes.
- Refer Denise to psychological care to teach her better strategies to deal with stress and worry. (Worrying directly depletes digestive function.)
- Eliminate foods that Denise negatively reacts to. (While food

sensitivities for each patient are unique, the top five food sensitivities that cause a myriad of negative symptoms not often associated with food are wheat, dairy, eggs, corn, and soy.)

- Add sweet-natured foods into her diet that support the gastrointestinal tract, such as rice, oats, squash, and sweet potato.
- Determine other organ systems that may be involved, such as the liver, lungs, and heart. (A well-trained TCM practitioner discerns other organ involvement and treats accordingly.)
- Refer Denise to supportive therapies, such as acupuncture, chiropractic, massage, and homeopathy, that will help her body return to a state of homeostasis by encouraging inherent self-healing mechanisms.

This approach to Denise's depression allowed her body to begin functioning more optimally, her hormones became better balanced, her energy increased, and she was able to engage in her life at a more pleasurable level. While her main underlying cause of depression was her weak digestion, someone else's could be completely different, which is why prescribing an antidepressant is an incomplete and inefficient treatment method. It is appropriate to fully consider potential root causes of any disease.

It is important to note that Denise's relief from depression did not happen overnight. It required a dedicated and involved approach from her as well as that of her health care team. Over time, her symptoms became less severe and less frequent. Sometimes, over the course of her treatment plan, her progress seemed slow.

I shared with Denise one of my favorite analogies, that of the rose. If you were to sit and stare at a rose blossoming, it would blossom so slowly that you could not even see the petals unfolding. However, if you step away and come back a couple of days later, you would see that the rose had indeed blossomed. When you *are* the rose, it is hard to step away and notice improvements in your health. It is important to take a moment and remember where you were just a few months prior. From this place, you may more easily recognize that while you haven't met your health goals yet, certainly you are closer than you were. Sometimes I get so involved in my patients' care that even I have to remind myself to be patient with the healing process.

Musculoskeletal Pain

Patients who have an injury that seems like it is taking forever to heal likely have tried several treatment options to little or no avail. Patients who are not healing as well or as quickly as desired commonly share the characteristic of dryness in their systems. More specifically, the fascia, the connective tissue surrounding organs and muscles, is dry, brittle, and lacking in flexibility.

DRYNESS IN THE BODY

I often liken the musculoskeletal system to a tree: A tree that is well nourished has strength by virtue of its flexibility. When the wind blows, the branches sway in all their glory. However, when the wind blows through a tree that is malnourished and dry, its branches splinter and break in response.

If your body is like a dry tree, you likely suffer from a stubborn version of some of the following conditions:

- tendonitis
- carpal tunnel
- sciatica
- plantar fasciitis
- hamstring strain

- chronic neck pain
- rotator cuff problems
- bursitis

People with a naturally long and lean frame are prone to dryness, although there are many things that make the fascia dry in the first place. Internal dryness can be influenced by hormone fluctuations, especially a decrease in estrogen in women, overwork, overthinking, general lack of rest and self-care, and not eating enough nourishing foods.

The key to helping soft tissues heal and be more responsive to treatment is to moisten and lubricate the fascia. I often recommend eating foods that act to nourish and moisten the body. These foods are slippery in nature and include asparagus, eggs, seeds, okra, and millet. It is also appropriate to avoid substances that dry out the system, which tend to be hot in nature. The biggest offenders are coffee (caffeinated or decaffeinated), alcohol, and non-steroidal anti-inflammatory drugs (NSAIDS). Receiving treatments that increase blood circulation, such as acupuncture, chiropractic, and massage, can also help internal dryness. Chinese herbs, when prescribed correctly by a practitioner with proper training in Chinese herbology, can be very helpful.

Still, to really and truly balance internal dryness, patients must adopt a routine of self-care that literally nourishes the body. Otherwise, they can eat a lot of moistening foods, take moistening herbs, and get lots of massage, acupuncture, and chiropractic care and still find that their bodies are slow to respond.

If you are lacking in the self-care department, you likely have one of two general habits: (1) overworking, overworrying, and over-exercising while not eating properly to nourish the body and not resting enough for proper restoration and healing to occur; and (2) under-exercising and eating foods that lack nourishment. Receiving counseling can be a helpful adjunct to the treatment plan if you are at this point.

What really scares me is how often patients have surgery to try to fix a problem when they suffer from poor self-care. If your body has trouble healing and your fascia tears easily, surgical intervention is not ideal. Surgery cuts right through the fascia and introduces another injury for the body to try to heal. For this reason, nourishing the fascia before surgery is a good idea.

The next time you find yourself complaining that you are not getting better, and you have tried everything and gotten no results, ask yourself about the condition of your general health. Make the commitment to improve your overall health, find out how to do so by consulting with integrative health practitioners, and get after it. It is up to you to change it. Will it happen overnight? Of course not. No drug or surgery will help you heal any faster, either. When you have a personalized treatment plan and a health care team that has your best interests at heart, you will eventually wake up feeling better.

> *"Good health is not something to take for granted;*
> *it is something we all have to work at to maintain."*
> —Elise P., teacher

CHAPTER 11

Take Back Your Health Care Power

Health care reform has been at the center of many political controversies. What is missing from both sides of the aisle is the idea that it is up to us as health care consumers to ensure that we are receiving the best care possible.

It is important to shift our thinking about what it means to maintain health. Asking questions and being active participants in the quest for wellness is essential. Instead of accepting the advice and prescription for care from your doctors and other health care providers, give serious consideration as to whether or not the recommended treatment approach makes sense to you as a patient.

Furthermore, too often we look outside of ourselves for answers to the health care system. The truth is, it is up to us change the state of our health care system. Once we shift the responsibility of our health away from health insurance and pharmaceutical companies to ourselves, we can take back our power to achieving and maintaining good health.

Perhaps you think this proposal is just plain absurd, wondering where you would find the wisdom and money to take responsibility for your health. But in reality, it doesn't take any more money to achieve health than it does to achieve illness, and it certainly takes more money to recover from being sick than it does to stay well.

When you decide to address your health at the grassroots level, you will find yourself making everyday choices that increase the odds of achieving and maintaining your health. To show my point, consider the following ideas for how you can increase the odds of achieving your best health, and therefore your best life, possible:

1. Explore health care options that are outside of the pharmaceutical realm, and think about when you are willing to accept pharmacological help (and the associated side effects) and when you are not. You are the one who gets to decide how you want to manage your health.

2. Accept the fact that your emotions affect your physical health, and vice versa. When we recognize that emotions and physical health are inextricably linked, we become open to the possibility of solving a health imbalance for good through a multidisciplinary approach. We can then stop covering up symptoms with a drug.

3. Give some thought to what it means to be proactive in maintaining your health. True preventive care means learning to pay attention to the clues your body and emotions give you to keep your health within the boundaries of wellness. These clues come in the form of symptoms and your intuitive sense. Don't wait until an illness shows up before you start doing something about your health. Disease is the result of a longstanding imbalance in your body, mind, and spirit.

4. Educate yourself about which foods nourish your body the best. There is not a one-size-fits-all diet plan. That said, there are certain items offered at grocery stores and restaurants that are unhealthy for

everyone because they are toxic. When reading labels to find out if a food is toxic or not, the general concept is that the more ingredients on the label, especially if they are chemically based, the less close to nature the food is and therefore the more toxic. Watch for artificial sweeteners such Splenda, Truvia, aspartame, and phenylalanine and artificial colors such as Red #40 and Yellow #7.

5. Realize that every single physical movement you make benefits your health. Every time you walk to the restroom, reach up in the cupboard, go for a walk, do some stretches, engage in strength training, do yoga, or go for a run, you are serving yourself in an important way.

6. Think of achieving and maintaining health as a journey. There are no shortcuts or quick fixes.

7. Believe your body has the inherent desire and ability to heal itself.

8. Stop making excuses. Choose to pay attention to the symptoms your body, mind, and spirit are providing to guide you to better health. Make the choice to explore the reasons for your health issues and the health care options that are right for you.

I realize that we as health care consumers are confused and have lost perspective on what we can do for ourselves to be well. I commonly see patients with the following conditions treated effectively without pharmaceutical drugs and other expensive allopathic methods of care:

- nerve pain
- restless leg syndrome
- peripheral neuropathy
- fibromyalgia

- chronic pain
- mild to moderate depression
- anxiety
- autoimmune diseases
- joint pain and stiffness
- injuries
- infertility
- blood sugar regulation
- weight issues
- headaches and migraines
- sinus problems
- allergies
- skin conditions
- fatigue
- insomnia
- acid reflux
- hormonal imbalances
- psychological distress and disorders
- irritable bowel syndrome
- constipation and diarrhea

There is tremendous hope for our health and health care system when we accept personal responsibility. When we open our eyes to the health care possibilities that lay outside of pharmaceutical drugs and what insurance will pay for, we create opportunities to fix underlying imbalances that cause disease. You can do this for yourself, and practitioners like me can help guide you when you are ready.

In the hospital setting, matters are heartbreakingly worse. If you or a family member has been admitted to the hospital, you will likely relate to the isolating, disjointed, and uncomfortable feeling that slowly resolves only after being released. When you are admitted to the hospital, too often you are nothing more than a number: a room number, a patient number, and numbers on a computer screen describing what the test results show. Your doctors may not be communicating, with you or each other. The doctor of the day sometimes does not even know why you are in the hospital. Your doctor often does not know your goal beyond whether or not you want life-saving measures should your heart stop while you are admitted.

It is imperative that you make your doctor aware of your health when you talk him or her. You can help yourself and your doctor by asking the following specific questions:

1. Is the suggested treatment plan wise for other aspects of my health? For example, if steroid shots are suggested, will they affect blood sugar safely? If surgery is recommended, can my body tolerate the recovery process, or would certain steps be necessary to help the recovery process go more smoothly?

2. What other body parts may be affected by the procedure and the recovery process? (The body compensates for a weak body part by affecting other areas of the body. What would your doctor recommend to ameliorate, or ease, those potential side effects?)

3. What can I do to prevent repercussions from the procedure you are recommending? Would physical therapy or massage therapy be helpful? Is it okay to take Chinese herbs or homeopathy for pain? (Painkiller medications are not one-size-fits-all because of a patient's pain tolerance, history with medications, and general preference. You should have several options available that align with your wishes.)

4. What nutrition will be necessary to help me heal? (Depending on your constitution, some foods will be better to speed the healing process than others. For example, if you are a menstruating woman who tends to be anemic, you will require more blood-nourishing foods such as red meat, beets, eggs, and dark-green leafy vegetables.)

5. What complementary therapies can help me heal faster and prevent post-surgical complications? (Acupuncture before and after surgery can enhance surgical outcomes by helping you healing faster. Homeopathy, medical massage, and chiropractic care can also help. Knee-replacement patients tend to get off pain medications and achieve their desired range of motion fairly quickly.)

6. Is my treatment plan going to be life-altering? (Changes in health can be stressful and hard to know how to handle. Life or health coaching or counseling may be helpful to make transitions less stressful.)

 It is unreasonable to expect just one or two doctors to carry the entire load of your care. Receiving adjunctive treatment from acupuncturists, massage therapists, chiropractors, and psychologists or counselors can be helpful to alleviate the chief complaint altogether. These modalities may also be used in combination with the care plan provided by a specialist.
 You may be thinking that all of this sounds great but that most insurance companies do not pay for nutrition consults, acupuncture, massage, chiropractic, and other modalities outside of conventional Western care. This may or may not be true, but what do you value most? How important is it to you to be healthy? Are you willing to risk your health by depending strictly on what the government or your insurance company is willing to pay for?

Take charge of your health and save your life *now*, and get it where you want it to be. You are the director of your health care journey. It is up to you to advocate for yourself and to refuse to accept less than the very best.

> *"After I had facial reconstructive surgery, the healing process was slow and frustrating. I was also facing the possibility of having more extensive surgery to attempt to fix issues I had from the first surgery, which included my eyes not being able to close all the way. I asked Dr. Schulte if she thought she could help, and she was confident that I would see an improvement in my healing. After several weeks of acupuncture therapy combined with massage and chiropractic care, my healing process was making much better progress, and the function of both my eyelids and my appearance improved dramatically Dr. Schulte had proven to be correct in her assessment.*
> *In fact, the treatment strategy exceeded both my and my surgeon's expectations. I quote the surgeon when he said that he was "amazed" at the improvement."*
> —Roger S.

CHAPTER 12
The Staggering Costs of Health Care

The high cost of health care has been widely acknowledged by government officials and the medical establishment. Whether healthy or ill, insured or uninsured, for health care reform or against it, most people want to live life as healthy as possible and would prefer to use their financial resources for more enjoyable options than sick care. The good news is that you can reduce health care costs while increasing your potential for vibrant health when you actively make conscious choices to maintain your health.

Stay healthy. Sounds simple, doesn't it? I have treated thousands of patients, so I know that maintaining and achieving health is not as simple as eating broccoli and taking nightly walks (although both go a long way toward helping).

I know that our emotional, mental, and physical health is entwined. I know from my own personal health care experiences that we are not the most objective guides of our own care when we don't have the help of an objective professional or group of professionals. We are often simply too emotionally connected to how we feel, in too much pain, or enduring too much suffering to make rational health care decisions for ourselves. This is why developing a relationship with a team of health care professionals whom you can trust is of utmost importance.

To help you determine whether investing your own money in your health care process is worth it, ask yourself these questions: If someone asked you to invest a bit of your money in the wisest way you could think of, how would you invest it? Would you invest in the stock market or an educational plan for your children or grandchildren? Would you upgrade your vehicle? Would you pay ahead on your mortgage? Would you get an MRI for clues to why you are experiencing pain? Would you spend it on medications such as antidepressants, antihistamines, and pain pills that you may not actually need? Or, if you knew that for a relatively low cost you could drastically improve your mental, emotional, and physical health and achieve the healthiest life possible, would you choose *you*?

What does it mean to invest in yourself? It means putting each aspect of your health and wellness first so that you can live your life in a way that serves you best. One common condition for treatment success is gaining the understanding that nothing and no one is more important than you are, yet learning to put yourself first can be an involved process. Often, the first step is to develop the belief that you are worth it. Putting yourself first can start with something as small as choosing a leisurely stroll at sunset instead of attending to a chore inside the house. Making an effort to engage in the benefits of addressing your health can be a giant leap forward in making a strong investment in both your health and your fiscal future.

> "Unfortunately, Medicare and other health insurances have not recognized how much money could be saved by encouraging patients to receive therapies like acupuncture. I have been willing to invest in my own care with my own money."
> —Ginny, retired teacher and school principal

CHAPTER 13
A Dying Patient's Perspective on Integrated Health Solutions

In Traditional Chinese Medicine, it is said that death occurs when the yin and the yang separate. During my time in practice, I have had the honor of sitting at the bedside of many of my patients as they actively die from chronic diseases such as cancer and pulmonary diseases. I am blessed to have had the opportunity to be a part of their dying process because I have partaken in a caring, compassionate, and involved approach to help these patients live their best lives possible while still on Earth.

Ginny's Story

I would like to tell you Ginny's story. Ginny, a seventy-three-year-old woman who was my patient for many years, passed away after a seven-year journey with stage 3C primary peritoneal carcinoma, an extremely rare cancer that looks and is treated like ovarian cancer. When Ginny heard the news of her cancer and looked up her diagnosis on the internet, she read the dire prognosis that the disease is 100 percent fatal.

The idea to voice-record Ginny's story came to me after I pondered something she had said when she knew that death was imminent. She said, "I'm not afraid of death, but I love life." She allowed me to record her story as she lay in her hospice bed, sharing poignant aspects of her care in a way that encompasses the main messages in this book. When I asked if I could share her story with my readers, she was more than happy to oblige. Hearing her perspective of integrative medicine as she approached the end of her life was a tremendous gift.

It was July 4, 2018. Ginny's chiropractor, Dr. Joseph Heinecke, and I had visited her in the local hospice care center the day before. Ginny had been admitted with the idea that she had only three to five days left to live. However, she proved the doctors wrong, and it was likely that she would be released from the care center later that week. I resolved to come back that day and give her an acupuncture treatment before her release, as her coming to the clinic was uncertain given that her home was an hour and a half away from Grand Junction. After celebrating Independence Day with my family, I returned to the care center to give Ginny an acupuncture treatment and record her testimonial.

Ginny helped me prepare her hospice center room for acupuncture by dimming the lights and organizing her bed in such a way that she would be comfortable. It was obvious she was an acupuncture veteran. I always have my acupuncture treatment rooms tidy, comfortable, and immersed in peaceful energy. It was almost as if Ginny knew that these were the conditions for this acupuncture treatment, as well.

As I inserted the needles, we began our recorded conversation with me asking her to imagine that the food she had been ingesting, now limited to liquids, would feed her healthy cells. Then she began to tell her story. I was captivated as she spoke, because even though it had been made clear to her that she was actively dying, Ginny remained focused on still being *alive*. Her yin was still feeding her yang, and vice versa.

Ginny recalled the first time she saw me at Healing Horizons. She had been referred by her oncologist for me to address her peripheral neuropathy, a painful and function-limiting condition that is often a side effect of taking chemotherapy.

When I met Ginny, she had already endured several rounds of powerful chemotherapy followed by a massive surgery. She was left with the peripheral neuropathy, which she described as feeling like she was walking on hot coals. After a brief course of acupuncture treatment, Ginny's peripheral neuropathy completely resolved, and her function was fully restored. She said, "That made me a believer." This success encouraged her to continue acupuncture to support her immune system so it could prevent recurrence of the disease. She regularly made the ninety-minute drive from her home to the clinic with her husband, Bob (who also became a patient), to seek acupuncture care.

Ginny said that the cancer remained in remission for five "wonderful" years, and she had maintained her TCM care for most of that time. The treatments served to boost her immune system, improve digestion, relieve stress, and address periodic body pain. However, the cancer recurred after a tremendously stressful year, when she had to contend with the deaths of both her mother and Bob's mother. Along with experiencing the grief of losing their moms, as the eldest of their siblings, both Ginny and Bob were left with the responsibility of handling the estates. Ginny said, "As I look back now, the one thing that happened in addition to the stress is that I did not make the time to fit in my regular acupuncture treatments."

I remember when Ginny and Bob were in the thick of that stress and the traveling required of them. I could feel a pulling and nagging sensation inside myself; it was my intuition, telling me they both needed care. As is so often the case, my urgings to them to engage in self-care fell short of the pressure the two were experiencing at the time.

When Ginny made it back in for care at the beginning of 2016, she said she was feeling something abnormal and asked me to palpate her abdomen. Cancer patients are often alarmed at every little lump or bump or unusual symptom. More often than not, these lumps and bumps and unusual symptoms are benign, but this time I felt a grape-sized lump, which I found concerning. I urged Ginny to see her oncologist.

A CT scan revealed a tumor in her abdomen, which was colon cancer, a secondary cancer of the original diagnosis. Ginny again underwent surgery and endured another round of chemotherapy, during which she developed an allergy to one of the drugs used in the treatment. The cancer then grew to include massive tumors in the vaginal wall and caused vaginal bleeding. She underwent twenty-five rounds of radiation accompanied by more chemotherapy. Remarkably, the acupuncture, which I had done on an acupuncture point on one of her big toes, significantly slowed the vaginal bleeding and again helped Ginny with neuropathy and maintaining her appetite and energy levels. Unfortunately, a later CT scan showed little reduction in her tumor growth.

At this point in her care, Ginny had developed debilitating pain in both of her hips that radiated down her legs. Her weekly acupuncture treatments were helping, but I suspected subluxation in her spine was contributing to her pain, and I knew that chiropractic would provide a beneficial adjunctive treatment to help alleviate the pain more effectively. That is when I referred her to a chiropractor.

Convincing Ginny to receive chiropractic care was no easy task, because she had heard negative myths surrounding chiropractic care. Even though she was hesitant, she was in enough pain to give chiropractic a try, especially as I assured her that I had a strong working relationship with the chiropractor I was referring her to. I also assured her that he and I would work together.

The chiropractic, in conjunction with the acupuncture, completely resolved Ginny's hip pain. The chiropractor's impression of the causes of her pain helped guide my acupuncture treatments. Ginny said she was grateful that she added chiropractic care to her treatment regimen, and she now viewed chiropractic as an "addition of activation of my nervous system. I found that as long as I continued my regular treatment regimen, I was able to buy myself more time."

Ginny's persistence and love of life kept her fighting. However, she soon learned that the cancer had metastasized to her liver and bloodstream, making any surgical efforts moot. Her oncologists and surgeons encouraged her to choose quality of life over last-ditch medical efforts that would likely make her miserable. She chose to continue chemotherapy, however, and went on to meet various goals in her life, including connecting with family, especially her grandchildren, whom she had always held close to her heart.

Ginny asked her oncology care team what to expect in the future. They let her know that she would eventually experience a small-bowel obstruction, which would signify that the end was near. Indeed, she soon began to experience bowel obstructions, which caused excruciating pain. Her medical teams managed the pain by pumping out the contents of her gastrointestinal tract and prescribing pain medication. Eventually, she had a feeding tube implanted, which extended her life further.

Ginny credited acupuncture as one of the main reasons she survived the original diagnosis by more than seven years. She said, "The one thing that has been a common thread throughout the entire last seven and a half years has been my regular acupuncture. Everything went well as long as I was able to make that a weekly priority."

As my interview with Ginny progressed, she displayed her role as her husband's wife, the protector of his heart. She had also been the protector of his health. She said, "It is hard for Bob to trust anyone. He is a private person, yet he feels comfortable seeing you and coming to you for help. That gives me more peace than you know." I have had the blessing and honor of getting to know Bob over the years of treating Ginny and then Bob himself.

Developing strong relationships—that is where superior health care lies. Because of the relationship Ginny and I had established, I was able to provide the next step in her care, which was to give her a sense of calm, as she was nervous to leave her family behind. Ginny said, "It gives me such peace that you know Bob and you know our story; he will not have to retell it because you already know." It is my honor to continue to provide the best care possible for Bob.

Ginny eventually made her last visit to Healing Horizons. She arrived emaciated, her cheeks sunken in and the gleam in her eyes fading. Sitting in the waiting room, she brightened a bit as she saw me walking toward her to take her to a treatment room. This time, I chose a treatment room near the room in which she would receive her chiropractic care after acupuncture.

We slowly strolled down the hallway, and just as we entered the treatment room, she collapsed into a sob. "I've lost four more pounds this week." She said that her appetite had disappeared and that she had to tell herself to take in nutrients. I asked her if this process of her body shutting down was harder than she had expected. She answered that she had been so used to being the strong one and that the weakness was overwhelming.

We managed to get her on the treatment table, where I proceeded to give her one last acupuncture treatment. During this time, her emotions were clearly prominent, likely contributing to her physical symptoms. She said she felt like she was letting her loved ones down.

With no time to refer Ginny to counseling, I was myself in the role of counselor. I reminded her of her strength. It was she who had outlived her prognosis arguably by seven years by advocating for her own health. It was she who had instilled strength and values in her children and grandchildren. It was she who loved Bob unconditionally and had been his partner since they were in college. It was she who touched the lives of thousands of children as a teacher and school principal.

After her acupuncture treatment, I found her chiropractor, Dr. Heinecke, who would see her next, and communicated Ginny's current state. I shared the ins and outs of her physical condition and added, "Anything you can do to help her release the guilt she is feeling for dying would be helpful." (Some chiropractors, like Dr. Heinecke, utilize a method called neuro-emotional technique, a mind-body approach to addressing physiological responses to stress.)

After the chiropractic session, I reunited with Ginny and Bob in the waiting room. She and I embraced, and as we hugged, she whispered in my ear, "April, you have been with me for seven and a half years. I'm so grateful. Thank you." I thanked her in return. As tears gently caressed each of our faces, I thanked her for the honor of serving as one of her health care providers and let her know how much she had taught me throughout the years. I then opened the clinic door, and she and Bob exited to their vehicle.

Later that evening, I was reflecting on my own emotions from Ginny's last visit when I realized why I was so emotional: after she and I and the rest of her healing team had spent years integrating yin and yang, I was witnessing the yin and the yang separating in her body. Ginny was a strong and vibrant woman. She lived life according to her values, and her passions guided her to live life to its fullest.

Traits of Healthy Patients

Patients who direct their own health care, like Ginny did, have several significant traits in common that lead to living a healthy life. They intuitively listen to their bodies and the clues their bodies provide in the form of emotional and physical symptoms. With that, they ask family, friends, and health care providers for referrals to doctors and other healing professionals with whom they may find successful treatment outcomes. They choose health care providers who align with their own value system. In other words, they deeply connect with their healing team.

Patients like Ginny do not settle for what anyone tells them when it comes to the state of their health, and they especially do not settle for poor communication between themselves and their healing team or among the health care providers themselves. If they have a question regarding a diagnosis or receive conflicted advice from their health care team, they seek out the answer that aligns with what feels right to them.

They also are willing to invest financially in their health with the full intention to be active participants in their health care journeys. Certainly, they do not allow the government or pharmaceutical companies to take charge of what is right or wrong when it comes to their bodies. Finally, they learn that caring for themselves means having self-love. Self-love means making the choice to put your health first by tending to your needs on every level, mental, emotional, physical, and spiritual, because your health is in your hands.

Mind Your Body and Your Spirit Will Follow

As a society, we have fallen prey to the idea of the cookie-cutter pharmaceutical approach to health care. We can do so much better than that. Take the power of your health back! Demand that your health care providers think about how the mental, emotional, physical, and spiritual aspects of your health are interconnected, and then ask for their guidance on how to treat your health care concerns as a whole picture. Encourage them to communicate with each other to meet your individual needs as their patient. Expect more. Demand more. Take charge of your health *now*.

Do not settle for the status quo. Take control of your health, and demand the opportunity to achieve true health and well-being so that you can enjoy your life to its fullest. Accept only the best health care you can find, and be willing to do the legwork yourself to achieve the healthiest you possible. Listen to your body, and then follow through on what it is requesting of you. Your body gives you clues in each moment of each day to guide you to a healthier and more fulfilling life. Choose you. Save your life now. You are worth it!

Index

Page references in italics indicate illustrations and t *indicates a table.*

acid reflux, 67
acupuncture
   for addiction, 62
   for anxiety, 117
   how it works, 60
   medical issues addressed by, 59
   origins of, 58–59
   for pain relief, 49, 59
   for peripheral neuropathy, 137
   psychology combined with, 51–52, 64–65
   qi unblocked by, 59
   relaxation during, 60, 62
   for sinus problems, 82
   for stress, 62, 117
   studies of, 54, 59–60
   for tremors, 53
addiction, 62
allergies, springtime, 34
allopathy. *See* conventional Western medicine
alternative medicine, 47n

American College of Preventive Medicine, 12–13
anger, 84, 87, 90
antibiotics, 76
antidepressants, 63, 102, 119–20
anxiety, 115–19
arthritis, 40, 68
The Art of Extreme Self-Care (Richardson), 105

back pain, 77, 113
balance
   case study, 108–9
   and the Healing Horizons Wellness Accumulation Program, 112–14
   overview, 107
   pottery analogy, 109–10
   sphere of health, 110–12
   symptoms as clues to imbalance, 14
bladder, urinary, 32t, 37, 38t, 85
blood, 15, 28–29, 30, 41, 88
body, mind, and spirit connection, 19–23, 142–43
body alignment, 76–77

bodywork/massage, 76–80, 118
bowel movements, 101–2

cancer case study, 135–41
candida, 70, 72
Centers for Disease Control and Prevention, 119
chicken soup for a cold, 41
Chinese herbs, 60–61, 123
Chinese medicine. *See* Traditional Chinese Medicine
chiropractic care, 66–67, 138–39, 141
chronic illnesses, healing from, 95–98
cognitive behavioral therapy (CBT), 117
coherence, 65
coldness, 39
colds, 41, 69
complementary medicine, 47, 53
Complementary Therapies in Medicine, 10–11
conventional Western medicine (allopathy)
boxed-in thinking in, 7–9
and complementary care, 5
defined, 75
dependence on test results, 11–12
diagnostic aspect of, 76
and the limits of insurance coverage, 12
and the limits of science, 9–11
overview, 3–6, 76
pharmaceutical drugs used in, 5–7, 12 (*see also* pharmaceutical drugs)
preventive medicine, 12–15
quick fixes in, 16
vs. TCM, 10, 26
thinking outside of, 16–17
value of, 3–4

dampness, 40, 101–2, 104
darkness, 35
depression, 50, 116–22
diet drinks, 71
digestion, 29, *30*
bowel movements, 101–2
and dampness, 101–2, 104
and depression, 50
digestive distress, 100–101, 103–5
and earth, 100
gut microbes, 102, 120
and lack of stomach acid, 67
organs of (*see* spleen; stomach)
overview, 99
and serotonin, 102
supporting the digestive tract, 105–6, 121
dopamine, 70
drugs. *See* pharmaceutical drugs
dryness, 40–41, 122–24

earth, 37, 38, 38t, 71–72, 100
emotional freedom technique (EFT), 117
emotions, 83–94
anger and liver/gallbladder, 84, 87, 90

body affected by, 19, 22, 63, 83–84, 126
as chemical changes, 62–64
fear and kidneys/bladder, 85
grief and lungs/large intestine, 85
imbalances and organ dysfunction, 90–94, 94
joy and heart/small intestine, 85
and the liver, 87–90
organs associated with, 38t
overview, 83–84
and pain, 86–87
as a response to illness, 63–64
worry/overthinking and spleen/stomach, 85–86
exercises
"create your day" meditation, 119
emotions and pain, 87
time to think outside of conventional medicine, 16
your body is calling, 35
experiential therapies, 117
eye movement desensitization and reprocessing (EMDR), 117

fascia, 54, 60, 123–24
father-child symbology, 38–39
fear, 85
fire, 37, 38, 38t
five elements, 36, 37, 38t
food
for anxiety, 117–18
bitter, 68, 74
for colds, 69
cravings for, 69–74
for dryness, 123
education about, 126–27
hot, 68
as medicine, 67–69, 74, 117–18
for menopausal hot flashes, 69
of poor quality, digestion harmed by, 103
salty, 73
sensitivities to, 107–8, 120–21
sour, 74
spicy, 74
for stomach pain, 69
to support digestive function, 105, 121
sweet, 68, 70–73, 121
warm, 68
functional medicine, 80–82, 92

gallbladder, 32t, 37, 38t, 74, 84, 92
gastroesophageal reflux disease (GERD), 66–67
gastrointestinal (GI) disease, 99
generating and controlling cycle, 36–39, 37, 38t
GERD (gastroesophageal reflux disease), 66–67
grief, 55–56, 85

Hahnemann, Samuel, 75
Healing Horizons, 52, 54–55, 75, 112–14, 117
healing journey, 95–98
healing team, defined, 2
health care costs, 133–34
health care power, 125–31

accepting the emotion-health link, 126
attention to symptoms, 127
declining drugs, 126–28
food education, 126–27
and hospitalization, 128–30
and insurance coverage, 130
physical movement, 127
proactive health maintenance, 126
reforming the system, 125
taking control of your health, 142–43
traits of healthy patients, 141–42
health hole, climbing out of, 95–98
health savings accounts, 12
heart, 30, 32t, 37, 38t, 85
HeartMath biofeedback, 65
heat, 40
HELLP syndrome, 4
holistic medicine, 47n
homeopathy
belief in, 75
following traumatic events, 23
for grief, 56
history and theory of, 74
hospitalization, 128–30
hot flashes, 69
Huang Di Nei Jing, 29

immune system, 78
indigestion, 67
inflammation. *See* dampness
Institute of Functional Medicine, 80
insulin resistance, 70
insurance coverage, 12, 130

integrated health solutions, 115–24
for anxiety, 115–19
for depression, 116–22
a dying patient's perspective on, 135–41
for musculoskeletal pain, 122–24
integrative and collaborative medicine
benefits, 45–56
case study, 54–56
collaborative medicine, meaning/ characterization of, 49–50
complementary medicine, 47, 53
doctor-patient relationship, 45–46, 52–54
integrative medicine, meaning/ characterization of, 47–49
key elements to successful treatment, 50–52
overview, 45–46
therapies, 57–82 (*see also* acupuncture; conventional Western medicine; homeopathy; Traditional Chinese Medicine)
bodywork and massage, 76–80
Chinese herbs, 60–61, 123
chiropractic care, 66–67
food as medicine, 67–69, 74
food cravings, 69–74
functional medicine, 80–82, 92
overview, 57
psychological care, 62–66
jing, 29, *30*
joy, 85

Kalanithi, Paul, 45–46
kidneys, 32t, 37, 38t, 85, 104

Langevin, Helene, 59–60
large intestine, 32t, 37, 38t, 85
liver
 and blood, 30, 41, 88
 and emotions, 84, 87–90
 in the generating/controlling cycle, 37
 liver qi stagnation, 42, 84, 87–90, 102
 and wood, 38t, 41, 74
 as a yin organ, 32t
lungs, 30, 32t, 37, 38t, 55, 85
lymphatic function, 78–79

massage/bodywork, 76–80, 118
medications. *See* pharmaceutical drugs
meditation, 118–19
menopause, 69
menstrual cramps, 108–9
meridians (channels), 26–28, 60
metal, 37, 38, 38t
mind, body, and spirit connection, 19–23, 142–43
mother-child symbology, 38–39
mother-daughter relationship, 104–5

NADA protocol, 62
National Acupuncture Detoxification Association (NADA), 62

National Center for Complementary and Alternative Medicine, 10
National Institutes of Health (NIH), 10, 99
nervous system, 65, 79

Oregon College of Oriental Medicine, 61
organs. *See also specific organs*
 connection among, 13–14, 30, 36–39, 37, 38t
 dysfunction and emotional imbalances, 90–94, 94
 emotions associated with, 38t
 timing of qi flow in, 93, 94
 yin and yang, 32, 32t
osteoarthritis, 68
overthinking, 85–86, 103

pain
 back, 77, 113
 and emotions, 86–87
 musculoskeletal, 122–24
pharmaceutical drugs
 antidepressants, 63, 102, 119–20
 for anxiety, 116, 118
 Chinese herbs combined with, 61
 conditions treated without, 127–28
 for GERD, 66–67
 use in conventional medicine, 5–7, 12
plantar fasciitis, 21
post-traumatic stress disorder (PTSD), 62
posture, 79

preventive medicine, 12–15
productivity vs. rest/rejuvenation,
    33–34
psychology, 62–66
    accepting psychological care, 65–66
    acupuncture and TCM combined
        with, 51–52, 64–65
    PTSD (post-traumatic stress
        disorder), 62

qi (life force), 27–28, 31, 59, 85, 93,
    94, 103. *See also under* liver
qigong, 25

reductionist view of health, 8, 20
rheumatoid arthritis, 68
Richardson, Cheryl: *The Art of
    Extreme Self-Care*, 105
Rolf structural integration, 15, 77

science, limits of, 9–11
self-love, 142
serotonin, 102
small intestine, 32*t*, 37, 38*t*, 85
spirit, body, and mind connection,
    19–23, 142–43
spirit, meaning of, 20
spleen, 30, 32*t*, 37, 38*t*, 85–86, 100
SSRIs (selective serotonin reuptake
    inhibitors), 102
Statista, 6
stomach, 32*t*, 37, 38*t*, 67, 85–86,
    100
stress, 86, 104, 107–9, 117
sugar, 70, 72–73

sugar substitutes, 70–71, 127
summer heat, 40
supplements, digestive, 106
surgery, 124
sweeteners, artificial, 70–71, 127
sympathetic and parasympathetic
    nervous systems, 65
symptoms
    attention to, 127
    as clues to imbalance, 14
    at night, 36
    unexplained, drugs prescribed for, 63

TCM. *See* Traditional Chinese
    Medicine
tendonitis, 14–15
tension, 79
test results, conventional medicine's
    dependence on, 11–12
tongue, 90
toxins, 104, 126–27
Traditional Chinese Medicine
    (TCM), 25–43. *See also* qi
    blood, 15, 28–29, 30, 41
    Chinese herbs, 60–61, 123
    vs. conventional medicine, 10, 26
    digestion in, 29, 30 (*see also*
        digestion)
    five elements, 36, 37, 38*t* (*see also*
        earth; fire; metal; water; wood)
    food as medicine, 67–69 (*see also*
        food)
    generating and controlling cycle,
        36–39, 37, 38*t*
    history of, 58–59

jing, 29, *30*
meridians (channels), 26–28
overview, 25–27, 57–58
pathological factors, 39–42, 68
pathologies between organ relationships, 39 (*see also* coldness; dampness; dryness; heat; summer heat; wind)
practitioner training in, 61
as preventive medicine, 13
research funding for, 10
symbology in, 38–39
yin and yang, 27, *31*, 31–35, 32*t*
trust, 52

University of Arizona Center for Integrative Medicine, 47–48

visualization, 118

water, 37, 38, 38*t*
Western medicine. *See* conventional Western medicine
whole-systems research, 10–11
wind, 39–41
wood, 37, 38, 38*t*
worry, 85–86, 103, 108

yin and yang, 27, *31*, 31–35, 32*t*

About the Author

As a renowned leader in integrative and collaborative medicine, Dr. April Schulte empowers people to live their healthiest lives possible by helping them find long-lasting solutions to conditions such as anxiety, depression, chronic pain, autoimmune diseases and more.

Dr. Schulte is a doctor of acupuncture and Oriental medicine and owner and clinic director of Healing Horizons Integrated Health Solutions. She is passionate about sharing her powerful, innovative approach to healthcare through her new book, Save your Life Now, her "Health Matters" podcast and speaking.

Dr. Schulte's personal journey of overcoming multiple eating disorders, physical pain from her years as a professional dancer, infertility and hormone imbalances enables her to connect with her patients and followers in a relatable way. A proud wife and mother of twins, she enjoys hiking in the Colorado mountains with her family and friends and continues to enjoy her first passion in life as a dancer.

To learn more about Dr. Schulte and her revolutionary approach to integrative medicine, visit her website: www.draprilschulte.com.

Made in the USA
Las Vegas, NV
23 February 2021